Nutritional Therapy Guide for a CFS Diet ...how to eat yourself healthy again

Vol 2 Includes:

Principles of Cellular Nutrition

Guide to Using Herbal Based Nutrition Supplements

Essential Superfoods for a CFS Diet

Warren Tattersall & Helene Malmsio

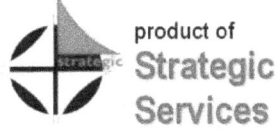

product of
Strategic
Services

The liability for damages, regardless of the form of the action, shall not exceed the actual fee paid for the product.

Contents

Introduction... 1

Chapter One: What is Chronic Fatigue Syndrome? *The Basics of this Condition*.. 3

Chapter Two: Therapies for CFS A Brief Introduction to Treatment Benefits........ 15

Chapter Three: Principles of Good Nutrition You May Not Be Getting as Much as You Think 31

Chapter Four: Cellular Nutrition From Your Plate to Your Cells................................... 43

Chapter Five: Supplements For A Healthy Villi How Using Herbal Supplements Helps Turn Around CFS   57

Chapter Six: Superfoods that Fight Chronic Fatigue Syndrome – and Provide Overall Wellness
.... 155

Conclusion - Handling Your Recovery... 203

About the Authors: 213

Introduction

Chronic Fatigue Syndrome has long been a condition on the edge of medical awareness. Many in the medical profession and much of the general public believed that it was not a genuine condition at all but something based out of lifestyle and mental state. Many believed that it was an excuse to avoid work or facing up to someone's personal situation.

This has changed now and the medical community and the general public see CFS as a medical condition but as there are no specific treatments people with CFS are very often told to just rest and eat well and that the condition will improve over time.

If you, or someone close to you, suffer with this condition then you will know that just waiting for eventual healing is not what you are looking for. You want a way to confront the problem and deal with it.

In this book we will explore what CFS is, how to identify it, and the medical and alternate treatments that are often applied to dealing with it. We will then look in depth at how you can use nutrition supplementation to assist with the problem,

Introduction

We will look at the history of people who suffer with CFS so you can see is one of those historic models fits your own situation.

We will then show you how to use nutrition supplements to deal with your condition and exactly what to expect when you use supplements; symptoms that you can expect to experience, how long you should expect before you see results, step-by-step through the recovery process and, ultimately, management processes once you are feeling well again to ensure that you do not relapse.

Chapter One:
What is Chronic Fatigue Syndrome?
The Basics of this Condition

Chronic Fatigue Syndrome, or CFS, is a condition that plagues millions of people worldwide. Imagine feeling as if you have the flu and have such fatigue that you're unable to carry out your normal activities. Worse, imagine being so fatigued all the time that you just cannot get up and function normally and you can only get out of bed for a couple of hours a day.

People all across the world are living with this condition. If you are one of them we hope we can guide you to be able to turn around your condition and to feel well again.

If you have someone you know who suffers with CFS, or has symptoms similar to the ones related here, then this book should give you an insight into their world, how they feel, and give you some practical strategies to help support them to deal with their condition.

What is Chronic Fatgiue Syndrome?

Normally, with CFS, when you go to the doctor, you don't have any specific illness that can be diagnosed and no one seems to understand how truly terrible you feel. Those who battle CFS can feel this way for months at a time.

In some cases the CFS condition seems to take over people's lives and they can lose not months, but years, of healthy living. These people are often young and often fit athletes and high performers in their field before they are stuck down by CFS.

In this section we'll outline some of the basic information about chronic fatigue symptoms and causes that are detailed further in the main body of this book, as well as the recommended methods of using nutritional therapy within a healing CFS diet.

CFS Symptoms

Chronic Fatigue Syndrome can be experienced in different ways. But the basic symptoms are:

Tiredness – extreme tiredness that isn't relieved after rest
Headaches – chronic headaches
Sleep problems – either you can't sleep or sleep doesn't bring rest
Muscle pain – pain that can't be explained by recent activities

These are the hallmark symptoms of the condition. But you may notice from this list that these symptoms could be part of other illnesses. It's important that if you suspect you have CFS that you speak with your doctor.

CFS is diagnosed if the above symptoms are present for a period of six months and there is an absence of another health condition. You'll need to make sure and rule out other illnesses that can cause these symptoms.

You may also experience other symptoms along with the main ones, including:

Food allergies and intolerances
Chronic tiredness that keeps people in bed much of the day and that requires regular naps to prevent the sufferer falling asleep as they try to undertake normal activities
Chronic diarrhea
Chronic sore throat
Night sweats
Weight loss
Nausea
Dizziness
Shortness of breath

For people with advanced CFS we do not need to list their symptoms as they are all too familiar with them but ultimately some people develop sensitivity to environmental conditions that can prevent them from living in normal modern society.

What is Chronic Fatgiue Syndrome?

Many other symptoms may apply to your specific case of Chronic Fatigue Syndrome. It's important to remember that this condition is very individual so you may have symptoms that others don't.

How Will CFS Impact Your Life?

Many people have trouble keeping up with their regular activities when they have CFS. You may feel like you just need to stay in bed and aren't able to go to work.

Many people find that they can't do many of the things they once enjoyed or that they cannot find the motivation to get started to get out undertaking these things. They just cannot get themselves moving.

What's worse, with CFS many people other people who see you with these symptoms don't understand that you have a real health condition. They may not understand why you can't work or they may feel frustrated that you're not able to continue old activities. This is often especially true for those who are closest to you.

Some people battle CFS for a few months and then get better, never having a relapse. But for many people there are cycles of fatigue followed by feeling better, then dealing with a frustrating return of fatigue.

Others seem to have these cycles but the fatigue level keeps getting deeper each time till they fall into a condition where they cannot even function in normal daily routines.

This can go on for a few years before the body is able to say goodbye to CFS and some people even deal with it over a lifetime. But with good therapy, particularly in the area of nutrition, you can turn around your condition and experience healing and once again feel better health.

What Causes CFS?

If you have chronic fatigue, you no doubt want to find out the cause. Unfortunately, there is no formal recognition of a specific cause of CFS yet. There are a few theories out there though:

The most common scientific theory is that CFS is caused by a virus that you've contracted at some point in your life.

We will talk later about the root cause potentially being an issue with your body's ingestion of nutrition. That is often brought on through lifestyle factors, high stress, and often seems to be linked to the use of antibiotics.

Others still seem to have a problem that has a foundation involving chemicals contamination and having residual chemicals in their body.

All of these paths to the condition seem to manifest in slightly different ways. The path out of them can also vary depending on the underlying issues but, in practical terms, the end result of how people feel and function when they are suffering with CFS seems to follow a similar pattern no matter what the cause.

Chronic Fatigue Syndrome has probably been around for centuries, but it's only been in the last century that it's gotten attention. And only in the last couple of decades has it been recognized as a true medical problem.

While CFS was once thought to be a psychological problem, in the past decade it's been seen by the medical community as a real illness. This has led to more research. While, as we said, there's no formally recognized cause yet, there are scientists hard at work looking to identify one and to better understand the condition.

The problem that faces people with CFS is that since no formally recognized cause has been identified this flows through to a situation where there isn't a medically recognized targeted medication, formalized treatment procedure, or cure for Chronic Fatigue Syndrome. It would be wonderful if you could get a prescription that would take care of CFS for good, but that's just not something available right now.

That is why this book covers alternative health information that does not claim to provide a cure but that has been shown to guide people back on to the path of healing and improved health.

We know that there are some things that can contribute to the development of CFS in the body as well as to other disease. Much of it has to do with our modern lifestyle and environmental stress that our lives place on us.

We expect that you will find some very logical and helpful answers for your own situation as we look at these things together and look at potential options, especially nutritional supplementation, to help deal with these things

For example, we're exposed to many more toxins nowadays than we have been exposed to in the past. Toxins can be found in the pollution in the air we breathe, contamination in the ground we walk on, and in more and more in the food that we eat. The more we're exposed to these toxins the more strain we place on the immune system.

In addition, the modern Western diet contains many processed grains and refined sugars that are also unhealthy for the body. And we don't get enough of the good, healthy foods we need.

Having a high stress lifestyle and broken sleep patterns can also cause the body to break down its immunity. A busy schedule coupled with lack enough sleep, or irregular sleep, can magnify the problem that stress creates for the body.

What is Chronic Fatgiue Syndrome?

We will look at how all these things can come together into a crisis for your body. This can lead to an event, or series of events, in life being a trigger point where people see their CFS condition as starting.

There are also more substances that are taken such as prescription medication, alcohol, and other illicit drugs that can break down your body's ability to fight infection and illness.

In thinking about your own lifestyle, you may be able to identify some factors that have led to your body's breakdown. But it's important not to dwell on the past and just make the decision to work at improvement from this day forward.

We will take time review the past with you though so you can see a path forward. We will then show you tools to deal with your situation and to get you moving back to health and to an active lifestyle.

Who Gets CFS?

Anyone can be diagnosed with Chronic Fatigue Syndrome. And even though there have been some cases in children, most are in either young adult age group (from 15 to early 20's) or older people between the ages of 35 and 50 years old.

A majority of cases of CFS appear to occur in women. In fact two thirds to three quarters of cases reported worldwide are women though there is a strong belief in medical circles that many CFS suffers never report it. It is likely that women are more likely to formally seek treatment rather than just trying to 'tough it out' as some men do.

There appears to be higher risk of CFS for people have a high stress lifestyle and that often includes high performers in fields from professionals to students and from business to elite athletes.

In the end, because there's no known cause it's hard to say who's at risk and who isn't. Anyone can get CFS.

Getting to a Diagnosis

As a starting point in dealing with CFS you need to know that you actually have the condition and that the symptoms are not actually there because you have a different conditional altogether.

That means medical diagnosis.

It's important in getting a proper diagnosis that you see the right doctor. While most doctors are now up to speed on Chronic Fatigue Syndrome, there are still very many who don't' understand it well or who don't consider that it is a serious medical condition.

Keep a journal of your symptoms to take with you to the doctor. Expect that you'll have to take a few blood tests so that the doctor can rule out other conditions that might possibly cause the symptoms you have.

What is Chronic Fatgiue Syndrome?

Once everything else is ruled out, you may be diagnosed with Chronic Fatigue Syndrome. At this point, talk with your doctor and see if he or she has treated patients with CFS before and how comfortable they are with alternative medicine practices.

If you feel like your doctor isn't listening to you or doesn't take your condition seriously, it's time to find a new one. You may get a good referral from someone in a CFS support group. Your own doctor may even suggest a practitioner that's better equipped to treat you.

In addition, you can contact your insurance company to see if they know of a doctor that specifically treats patients with CFS. Finding a good healthcare provider can help you to get better treatment so that your symptoms can be less problematic.

Will I Get Cured?

Once someone is diagnosed with CFS, searching for a cure is usually the first thing on his or her mind. Unfortunately, as we have said, there's no definitive medical cure for Chronic Fatigue Syndrome at this time.

In order to have a medical cure the condition, it would be necessary to know the cause. And since no single cause has been identified, there's no known medical cure. However, that doesn't mean that there's nothing you can do.

We are going to cover in detail in this book alternative health methods you can use to address your condition without drugs and medication. As a starting point though it is good to check all your options and to have as solid a foundation of knowledge about your condition as you can.

There are some medical interventions that can help you to have relief from symptoms such as joint pain and headache. You can also get prescription medication to help with depression that goes hand in hand with CFS.

In addition, some people choose to use prescription medication to help with sleep.

Medications like these can helpful for some people in the short term, and that's fine, but we expect you'll find that you get the most help from lifestyle changes and other therapies.

While there's no recognized cure for CFS, that shouldn't lead you down the road of feeling discouraged. The good news is that there's much you can do to help manage the symptoms and improve your immunity and energy levels.

In this guide you'll learn some basic information about CFS therapies and you'll learn more detailed information about how nutritional therapy can potentially give you control of your Chronic Fatigue Syndrome and allow you to get back to a fully active lifestyle.

No matter how badly you're feeling right now, you can have hope that it will get better with lifestyle and behavior intervention. We will show you step you can take to get relief from CFS and return to feelings of health and vitality.

Chapter Two:
Therapies for CFS
A Brief Introduction to
Treatment Benefits

There are many different ways you can work to treat Chronic Fatigue Syndrome and get your quality of life back. By getting help from professionals and making some lifestyle changes, you'll see improvement in your health, your energy levels and the strengthening of your immune system to be better able to resist the health problems that you are currently succumbing to.

We will start the more detailed look at options and treatments that people have been using over the years so you can see if there are answers there for your own situation.

These CFS treatments and self-help steps have been covered in great detail in our first book in this series, *"How to Beat Chronic Fatigue Syndrome...and get your life back!"* which also includes step-by-step instructions for how to implement them. You can read more about this book here:

http://www.amazon.com/Beat-Chronic-Fatigue-Syndrome-ebook/dp/B00ANM51XG

But to help you get at least a general overview of the most commonly recommended and recognized CFS therapies, we will give a brief outline the most prominent of them again in this book.

After that we will get on with the core purpose of this volume in the series, which is giving you a very in-depth look at the specific use of nutrition for designing a CFS diet to help you to eat yourself healthy again, including using natural supplements, exactly how to use them, and what to expect to experience when you do.

There is no doubt that learning the finer points of nutrition, how we digest our foods to get maximum benefit, and what foods give us the greatest results, is crucial to learning how to overcome the effects of chronic fatigue syndrome.

This should also give you a much deeper understanding and more control over how to help your body to help itself to heal. Once you have read this book you will definitely wish you had learned all this years ago!

But first, let's have a brief introductory look at some of the self-help steps and CFS therapies that you should be incorporating into your life if you are not already doing so.

Cognitive Behavioral Therapy

Cognitive Behavior Therapy (CBT) is a form of therapy that helps you learn to make changes in your behavior that will support your wellness. This therapy will help to change the way you think about your illness so that you can take more positive steps to improve your health.

Steps include keeping a Journal to pay attention to how you're feeling each day. This will help you to determine when you tend to have the most energy and when you're low on energy. Understanding this can help you to set out your day's activities effectively.

You'll then work to schedule your days so that you take advantage of peaks of energy and schedule rest periods for your low energy 'down times'. You'll be able to create a routine for your life that allows you to accomplish more than you ever could before.

Through work with a CBT therapist, you'll also learn to change your attitude. Many people with chronic illness develop an attitude of defeat from the constant plague of symptoms. While that's normal, you don't have to accept it. This state of exhaustion and feeling of hopelessness can spiral downward into a deep depression, so anything that can help you prevent slipping into chronic depression is good.

You can begin to see the good in your life and have a more positive attitude to help you get through the trying times of CFS flare-ups. Instead of what you don't have and can't do, you'll focus on what you can overcome and the good things you do have in your life and under your control.

You'll also learn to prioritize your tasks and what is truly important in your life, so that you don't waste energy on things that are unimportant and drain your energy needlessly. It's also helpful to learn how to be flexible so that even if you had something planned, you can listen to your body and make necessary changes when needed.

People who have CFS often have trouble focusing and concentrating on tasks for any time. Through CBT you'll also learn techniques to help you stay more alert and to be present in the moment.

Cognitive behavior therapy is a wonderful way to help you reframe your thoughts and feelings and learn to cope with the challenges of Chronic Fatigue Syndrome. When you participate in it you'll be able to improve the way you feel and to manage your schedule better.

Pacing

Pacing is a technique you often learn through cognitive behavioral therapy, but you don't have to participate in CBT to understand its principles. With CFS you'll notice that you do have some high energy days.

What normally happens is that when you have high energy, you try to compensate for all the days when you've had low energy levels. It's important to pace yourself so that you don't have even more fatigue later.

Pacing will keep you from using up all of your energy stores and allow you to have more good days than you would if you overexerted.

This strategy breaks down your days into chunks of activities interspersed with breaks to allow for rest and recovery between projects.

When you learn to implement this on a daily basis you will definitely benefit from more sustained energy, and will experience less breakdowns that need days or weeks of recovery time.

Physical Therapy

Exercise is actually beneficial for someone with Chronic Fatigue Syndrome. However, when you feel exhausted it might be the last thing on your list. With the help of a physical therapist you can develop a graded exercise program.

With this type of program you'll start very small. Perhaps you'll only exercise for five minutes a day at first. But you'll continue that program until you're not exhausted by the five minutes. Even when you have a high energy day, you'll stick to the short routine.

Once you've built up to a comfortable five minutes, you can add a few more minutes for the next week or two. You'll continue in this manner until you've reached an amount of time that makes sense for you.

It may seem overwhelming to exercise when you have CFS, but with the help of a physical therapist you'll be able to create a program that works. It will take effort and determination on your part, but the benefits will make the effort worthwhile.

Massage Therapy

Many people report feeling better when participating in massage therapy. Massage helps to release toxins from the soft tissues of the body. It also helps to provide relaxation and comfort for sore muscles.

If you're having trouble sleeping, massage can help your body to relax and get more rest. Swedish massage will give you that comfortable and relaxed feeling. If you want more energy, though, deep tissue massage will provide more benefits.

Massage is especially beneficial for people who are already suffering some of the common secondary health issues leading from CFS such as arthritis, rheumatoid arthritis, and general joint inflammation.

Chinese Medicine

Chinese medicine incorporates several methods such as herbal treatments, cupping, acupuncture, moxibustion and massage

In Chinese medicine diagnosis comes from discussions with the patient as well as an examination of the pulse and tongue.

This type of medicine has been around for many thousands of years and has given many people a great deal of improvement. Where Western medicine fails, Chinese medicine can often bring relief.

You can look for a practitioner of Chinese medicine in your area. You want to go beyond someone who took a weekend course on herbs or acupuncture and got a certificate. Look for a person with a doctorate in Chinese medicine or Oriental medicine.

This is more than just a few techniques, it's actually a philosophy about the body and how energy moves through it. It may seem unorthodox to you, but this type of medicine can be very beneficial to the body.

Therapies for CFS

Chiropractors

Chiropractors can work to help relieve some of the symptoms you feel from CFS and help improve your wellness. This type of doctor works to keep your skeleton in alignment.

By doing so, your nervous system is able to work properly. You don't have blockages between neurons or pinched nerves that can cause pain and discomfort.

Chiropractic care can help relieve muscle pain, headaches, and other CFS symptoms.

Chiropractic offices also tend to work with other alternative medicine practitioners such as acupuncturists, and kinesiologists. Chinese medicine practitioners, nutritionists, and massage therapists to create a wellness team for you.

Homeopathy

Homeopathic practitioners go beyond the boundaries of Western medicine to provide herbal and natural remedies. They may prescribe herbal formulas in the form of capsules, drops, or creams.

They work with you to discuss your needs and develop a treatment program that's tailored to you individually. Homeopathic practitioners should be highly trained and certified in your area.

Western Medicine Approaches

With Western medicine, there are some traditional treatment options that your doctor may offer you. While there are no medications specifically designed for Chronic Fatigue Syndrome, there are medications available that will relieve symptoms.

This type of therapy can get you through a CFS flare up until you feel improvement from the natural decline of the condition or from lifestyle changes and alternative treatments. Many people feel uncomfortable taking prescription medication long-term.

However, medication can be useful for many people who are experiencing problems. It's important to educate yourself about the possibilities you can expect from a traditional physician.

Sleeping Medications

Ironically, people who have CFS often have a hard time falling asleep. Medications to aid in sleep can help you to get some rest when you're unable to fall asleep on your own. It's important to realize, though, that these aren't meant to be taken long term.

Many sleep aids are habit forming, meaning that you become dependent on them to sleep. They're best used for short-term help.

Long term recovery of CFS requires learning the sleep hygiene and creating the sleep environment, which will enable consistent and restful sleep.

Antidepressants

Chronic Fatigue Syndrome also goes hand in hand with depression. Feeling badly and being unable to do the things you enjoy long-term can lead to depression that can be further debilitating.

Antidepressants can help to increase your brain's serotonin levels and improve your mood. They can take the edge off of the frustration that comes from chronic illness in your life.

They can also actually help with sleep as well. You may find that short term use of these medications may help you to improve your ability to face the challenges of CFS.

Anti-inflammatories

Anti-inflammatories are also helpful with reducing the inflammation in the body that is often associated with CFS. It can also help to relieve joint pain and make you more comfortable and able to perform daily tasks.

Some anti-inflammatories can be purchased over the counter while others require a prescription.

Learning the diet and nutrition changes that reduce inflammation in your system is definitely the preferred long-term method to achieve this result.

Gateway to More Services

If you have a physician that's fluent in working with Chronic Fatigue Syndrome, you may also take advantage of referral services. For example, your doctor can refer you to nutrition services, physical therapy, and even alternative medicine practices.

Medical doctors may not have all the answers, but they can provide help when you're experiencing symptoms.

Exercise

While physical therapists can help you to determine the perfect physical activity program, you don't have to go to therapy in order to add a little exercise into your life. Beginning a physical exercise program can be very beneficial to you.

Start wherever you are – in other words, don't try to run a marathon. If you're not active at all, try walking for two or three minutes each day. Do that whether you have high energy or low energy.

When you get to a point that it's always easy for you to complete the short increment of time, add another minute or two. In this way you can make exercise a part of your life even if you're very fatigued.

Therapies for CFS

Over time, you'll find that you feel more energized and that the exercise also benefits the muscle pain you've had.

Sleep

Sleep is necessary in order for your body to be rested and restored. In fact, not having enough sleep and regular sleep patterns may even be a contributing factor to developing a CFS condition.

But with CFS it can sometimes be difficult to get a good night's sleep. It's important that you set up a routine to help make it easier.

That may include eliminating caffeine and sugar – especially at night – and changing your bedroom environment to be more conducive to sleep. It's also important to go to bed and wake up at the same time each day.

Even if you're not tired, it helps to force yourself to get in bed to establish a routine. Eventually your body will follow.

You need eight to ten hours of sleep each night, especially when you are trying to recover from being unwell, so do the best you can to respect your body's needs.

You may also want to try a natural supplement called melatonin that can provide you with the chemical you need to get sleepy and stay asleep.

Stay Away from Addictive Substances

Habit forming substances such as alcohol and other drugs can really magnify CFS. When you have Chronic Fatigue Syndrome, you can't handle the strain that these chemicals place on your body.

Often people turn to this type of substance when they feel bad looking for a solution to their problems. Unfortunately, the addiction actually just makes the problem worse. Addictions aren't limited to drugs and alcohol.

Gambling, overeating, and smoking can also cause negative health consequences for you. It's important to pay attention to your behavior and determine if you have a problem in any of these areas. You may want to seek help if you find that your life is overcome by them.

Probiotics

We are inundated by antibiotics that have been overprescribed and have even made it to our food supply. It's important to make sure you introduce healthy bacteria to the body to keep things in balance.

There are many supplements that you can take to add healthy bacteria to your gut. You can also get probiotics from foods such as yogurt and kefir. This simple step can help your immune system to get stronger and can reduce inflammation in the body.

27

Therapies for CFS

Vitamins

There are several vitamins that support your immune system. You'll want to make sure you get plenty of vitamin C, vitamin E, and zinc. There are also supplements such as colloidal silver that have been known to improve CFS symptoms.

Omega 3 fish oil can also help to relieve the inflammation in the body as well as improve your mood. In fact, fish oil has been shown in some studies to be as effective as antidepressants.

In this volume of our CFS series you will learn all about this and how to get maximum benefit from both natural superfoods and from natural nutritional supplements that have been proven to work for both of us as well as the people we have worked with over the past 20 years.

Detoxification

We come in contact with all kinds of toxins in the environment and even in the food we eat. We also take in emotional toxins by being around people and situations that aren't good for us.

Purifying the body of toxins is one way to relieve the CFS symptoms. Far infrared saunas are tools that can help you to detoxify the body through perspiration. Massage can also release toxins.

When it comes to emotional toxins, it's important to avoid anything that brings negativity into your life. When you have a positive attitude and surround yourself with positive people and media you'll find that you feel better.

Nutrition is also very important for cleaning out toxins from the body and allowing nutrients to get into your cells. That will be the focus of the next chapter.

You can read the full process and the detailed steps to take for applying this range of CFS therapies in our first book of the series: **http://www.amazon.com/How-Beat-Chronic-Fatigue-Syndrome/dp/1481192914**

This volume 2 book in the series that you are reading now will focus on how your digestive system once it is compromised can hinder all and every attempt to deal with CFS, unless you help your body to heal on a cellular level and to repair its ability to digest and fully absorb the nutrition you are eating.

It is a surprisingly complex issue and not one that is easily fixed overnight. The information on using nutritional supplementation as a therapy requires you to evaluate your levels and causes of CFS to define what methods and quantities of supplements you will be working with when you eat yourself back to good health.

Therapies for CFS

At this point, let's begin with looking at what your ideal nutrition should look like, and why we so very rarely manage to get any real benefit from the foods we are eating – even including Superfoods!

Chapter Three:
Principles of Good Nutrition You May Not Be Getting as Much as You Think

As a starting point for wellness there is no question that nutrition is critical to good health. For vibrant health there is a need for top quality nutrition in a form that your body can absorb it and make use of it.

The saying "You are what you eat" couldn't be more true.

Your relationship with food is very intimate and when you don't have good nutrition, or don't have enough nutrition, or don't have the right nutrition, then your body suffers in many ways.

Many people think that they have a healthy diet, but are actually lacking some, if not many, of the nutrients they need. Many of these nutrients are ones that your body needs every day as it cannot produce them for itself.

It's important if you are going to get yourself to optimum health to first understand what nutrients are necessary for a healthy body and immune system.

Principles of Good Nutrition

Protein

Everything in the body is actually made of protein. In order for our bodies to have the building blocks needed to keep organs healthy and strong, it's necessary to eat protein every day.

Without enough protein, your body can't build muscle cells and can't maintain structures that are vital to you. Most people think of protein as coming from meat, but it can also be found in plant sources.

Think of the number of vegetarians and vegans who do not eat meat and it is clear that there are interesting and effective forms of protein from other sources.

Carbohydrates

Over the years carbohydrates have gotten a bad rap. The truth is that our bodies need carbohydrates in order to have a source of energy. When you deprive your body of carbs you actually harm it.

Your brain needs sugar in order to work properly and carbohydrates and the body's preferred source of energy.

If you don't get enough carbohydrates, you also become dehydrated.

The best carbohydrates come from fruits, vegetables, and whole grains. The carbohydrates that aren't good for the body come from processed grains, such as white flour, and refined sugars.

Many weight loss and other diet programs vilify carbohydrates, but carbohydrates aren't bad. Healthy carbohydrates are essential to maintaining good nutrition.

Fats and Oils

In the 90s, fat was a bad word. Many people began subscribing to a fat-free diet. This was when fat free products became all the rage and people counted fat grams vigilantly to lose weight.

But there has since been a backlash and we now know that fat is essential to good health. In fact, all those fat free products are actually worse for you than the full fat versions. Why is this?

In order to replace the flavor and satisfaction that comes from fat, many products simply substituted sugar.

This makes those products higher in calories that will eventually be stored as fat. If not sugar, flavor is added with artificial flavorings that are even worse for the body.

It's essential to get plenty of healthy fats from plant and fish sources. Olive oil, nuts, avocado, and fish oil all provide necessary monounsaturated fats that prevent heart disease and reduce inflammation in the body.

Fats also provide a concentrated amount of calories that help us to feel satisfied by foods. Oils also help lubricate the joints and help cells to remain structurally intact.

Fiber

Fiber is a type of carbohydrate that can't actually be broken down by the body. It works to pick up free cholesterol and keep it from becoming deposited in the blood vessels. Fiber also has benefits for digestive health.

Fiber works to bulk up waste so that you can have regular bowel movements. It also "scrubs" the intestines to keep things clean and prevent disease.

For over 20 years the Americian Medical Association (AMA) has said that up to 70% of bowel cancers could be avoided by the simple measures of adding more fiber to your diet and taking regular exercise.

This is one nutrient that most people are lacking because they don't eat enough whole grains, fruits, and vegetables.

Water

Most of your body is made of water. It's essential for your cells to have plenty of water in order to function properly.

Water is also a medium for removing toxins from the body and for lubricating the body.

By the time you feel thirst you're already way behind on your water intake. It's important that you drink plenty of water in order to have the best health possible.

And understand that tea, coffee, cola and other flavored and carbonated drinks, even most 'fruit juice drinks', are not a substitute for water when your body needs hydration.

This also does not mean that you have to force yourself to drink liters or gallons of water daily, it simply means that you need to make sure you drink at least 3-8 normal sized glasses of water and become more aware of the signs of your body becoming dehydrated so that you can learn how to prevent this happening.

Vitamins and Minerals

Within the food you eat are essential vitamins and minerals that each plays a part in the symphony that is your body. It's not necessary to talk about each one individually, but it's important to note that most people are vitamin deficient.

Most of this is a result of the processed foods that we consume rather than fresh, whole foods.

Principles of Good Nutrition

Botanical Factors

Your body also needs plant products: herbs and other living sources of nutrition's that cannot be found in other food groups.

A Junk Diet

You need to get all of the nutrients listed above very day in order for your body to repair cells that are injured and replace cells that are dying. Unfortunately, the modern diet in industrialized countries is sorely lacking in many nutrients.

The majority of people that consume the Western diet eat foods that are high in calories and low in nutrients and low in fiber. Refined sugars, white flour, and artificial chemicals are rampant in food on the supermarket shelves.

In study after study, it's shown that people eating a Western diet consume too much sugar, fat, and artificial chemicals and not enough water, fruits, vegetables, and whole grains. This alone can lead to poor nutrition. But this isn't the only problem.

Toxins in Our Food

Because of modern farming practices, even the fruits and vegetables that we have to choose from have been exposed to fertilizers and pesticides that are harmful. And recently genetically modified foods released on the market have caused alarm in the general population and also many scientific circles.

When it comes to meat, eggs, and dairy products we also have to pay attention to the use of hormones and antibiotics that go into the animals. These are designed to cut down on disease in overcrowded and unhealthy environments where animals are raised.

These hormones and toxins make their way into our bloodstreams through the food we eat and can cause problems.

Less Nutrition in Nutritious Foods

In the industrialized age we live in, fruits and vegetables that should be bursting with nutrition are often lacking. There are a few farming practices that make that happen. For example, seeds are often planted in soil that is low in nutrients.

This comes from over-farming an area of land and not practicing proper crop rotation or letting the field rest between crop seasons. This is all in the name of making more food at a cheaper price.

The problem is that plants get much of their nutrition from the soil. When the soil is already depleted and low in nutrition, the foods it produces are also lower in nutrition than they should be.

Principles of Good Nutrition

In addition, foods are also picked at the improper time. Many foods are picked before they're actually ripe so that they can be stored and shipped all over the world.

What that means for you, the consumer, is that the "fresh" food you pick up at your local market isn't always as nutritious as you'd like it to be.

While the produce may be cheaper than it would be if grown under proper local and seasonal conditions, you're also getting an inferior product that is force fed chemical nutrition and forced into ripening for out of season markets, including being gassed in some cases.

Your Healthy Diet May Not Be Healthy Enough

While it's certainly a good idea to have a diet high in all of the essential nutrients, the food you eat most likely in this day and age may not be enough. With low quality food being produced you may still not get what you need even if you eat the majority of your diet as healthy plant foods.

Many healthcare providers recommend that you at least take a regular multivitamin to supplement the nutrients you aren't getting from your food. But is that enough? It might not be if your body isn't prepared to absorb the nutrients you provide it with.

And there are so many products on the market that it can be very confusing to determine what product or popular brand is really going to help improve your wellness. It's important to understand nutrition at the cellular level to make a good choice. We'll discuss more about that in Chapter Four.

The Results of Poor Nutrition

Chronic Fatigue Syndrome is obviously exacerbated by poor nutrition. But there are many other health conditions that can result from not getting the right fuel for your body. The food we eat is like filling up on regular Unleaded gas when we need Premium.

People, even very young and seemingly healthy people, can have problems with low energy, problems with lack focus and attention, and immune deficiency. They may be more likely to feel the effects of stress as well.

And as you age, poor nutrition can lead to more serious conditions such as:

Diabetes
Heart disease
Cancer
Autoimmune diseases
Digestive issues
Hormonal issues
Depression
Stroke
Rapid aging

Principles of Good Nutrition

On the other hand, if you have the best possible nutrition combined with the right supplements, you can greatly improve your health.

You can have more energy, fewer problems with illness and disease, and even look better.

Modern Food Production is Related to Disease

Many people who have Chronic Fatigue Syndrome work hard to immediately improve their diets. This is a good thing. Unfortunately, the dramatic improvements you expect from a better diet are often not as impressive as you would expect from making such positive changes.

If you've been trying to eat a healthy diet, you're still doing the right thing. It can just be frustrating because it isn't enough to counteract all of the toxins and poor food production practices that lead to the deficient food we have today.

A hundred years ago people ate food they grew themselves or that was grown nearby in their local region. There weren't any laboratory made chemicals added to the soil or unhealthy fertilizers. Instead, people used what we now refer to as organic farming methods and they protected and cherished the farmland.

Food was full of important nutrients and you didn't see the problems we see now with obesity, diabetes, and other chronic diseases. With modern forced farming techniques, with fruits and vegetables often being picked before they have naturally ripened, with longer transport and storage practices, it's impossible today to get that same quality of nutrition from the food we eat unless we grow it all ourselves in an organic way.

Unfortunately, that's not a realistic choice for most people. Instead, we need to learn to work with what we do have. By eating the most healthful food possible and adding in high quality nutritional supplements, you can achieve better results.

However, since you cannot control all your food origins and storage to ensure you are getting the quality your body needs to recover and maintain good health, it makes good sense to enhance your daily nutrition efforts by including natural supplements in your CFS diet plan.

Herbal Based Nutritional Supplements

Herbal based nutritional supplements offer a solution to this modern day problem. For a relatively low cost, you get many added health benefits. These supplements are specially formulated to give nutrition to your body at the cellular level.

The supplements combine the technology of modern science with the wisdom of ancient herbal practices to develop a program that gives you the best of both worlds.

In order to truly understand how these supplements can support good nutrition, it's important to understand some basics about how the cells of the body are healed and replaced.

In the next chapter you'll learn some basic information about how we can cleanse the body of toxins to make room for nutrients to be able to make it to the right place. This is a system that's been interrupted by the impact of toxins in our food and environment, but there is a solution.

Chapter Four:
Cellular Nutrition
From Your Plate to Your
Cells

Eating seems like a pretty simple process. You start with a plate of food, eat it and process it through your digestive system. You ingest the food, the nutrients go where they're needed, and the waste is removed.

Basically this is correct, provided your body is working efficiently and, in truth, what goes on inside the body is much more complicated than it first appears to be.

In order for your body to really get the benefits from the food you eat it has to do three things.

First, your cells must be cleansed of toxins.

Second, your small intestine must be functioning efficiently and, for many of us, that means they need to be repaired.

And third, healthy cells are allowed to absorb nutrition.

This process can be complex and if your system is not currently working at full efficiency it requires that you have the right balance of nutrition and detoxifying agents to get things back in balance.

Cleaning Out the Toxins

When you eat a diet that's low in fiber and high in processed foods (typical of a Western diet) you actually slow down digestion. This causes food to begin to decompose in your gut rather than to be digested at a normal pace.

This process of decomposition causes the creation of toxic conditions in the body, in addition to the toxins that are already part of the food in the first place.

The liver's job in the body is to filter toxins and create bile to help break down fats. As you can imagine, a diet that's high in saturated fat and toxins will need to massively draw on the energy of the liver to break those toxins down and eliminate them from the body.

With the typical Western diet we put much more strain on the body than it's made to originally handle. Remember, only a century ago we were eating food that was produced locally from nutrient dense soil and had very little refining from its natural state prior to being eaten.

Dealing on a daily basis with over processed and toxin laden foods can cause the liver to become seriously enlarged and unhealthy. Anyone who suffers from a bloated liver or from gallstones can tell you in detail about how excruciating the pain is and how you normally end up in surgery to resolve the problem once the liver is terminally damaged.

This strain on your liver is bad enough, but other parts of the body are also affected. The poor foods we eat often require additional digestive enzymes in order to be broken down.

The pancreas is the organ in the body that's responsible for making those enzymes and it can also become enlarged. Incidentally, this is the organ that makes insulin.

Type 2 diabetes is a result of a pancreas that doesn't produce insulin that can be used by the body.

While the liver and pancreas help to produce chemicals that break down the foods we eat, the real job of absorbing nutrients goes to the small intestine.

It's here on the inside walls of the intestine that tiny fingerlike projections called villi, and upon them fine micro-villi, actually absorb nutrients from the food in our digestive system.

Those nutrients are then delivered via the bloodstream and lymph system throughout the body.

Poor nutrition and inflammation from toxins causes the villi to become brittle and break off. They can even be compressed in such a way that they aren't able to absorb nutrients.

This is called 'energetically impaired' villi and it means that even if you are eating excellent quality food, you will still not be capable of absorbing the nutrition from it that you should be getting.

While the body is very resilient and can handle most of our daily challenges under normal circumstances, the toxic diet can be too much for it to cope with over time.

In the short term this buildup of toxins can cause:

Diarrhea
Acne
Constipation
Body odor
Bad breath
Eczema

After years of abuse the body will finally begin to show the signs of wear and tear and you develop a greater risk of succumbing to serious illnesses such as cancer. Chronic Fatigue Syndrome may also be linked to this breakdown in your body's resistance and ability to fight back against life threatening diseases.

The good news is that you don't have to accept that this condition will occur in your body. Good quality nutritional supplement products not only provide powerful nutrition to assist your body to rebuild villi, they include herbs that are specifically known for detoxifying the body.

They do so in a way that's not painful or too shocking for your system, but they're quite effective. They cause the toxins to be removed from the tissues where they like to hide – in the muscles and organs.

Then those toxins are sent to the bloodstream where they can be eliminated by the kidneys through your urine. They are then no longer blocking your body's attempt to absorb nutrition from the food you are eating and the nutrition products are proving additional high quality nutrition that can also be effectively absorbed.

Another critical aspect of this sort of nutrition therapy is that you drink up to eight glasses of water so that you can provide a medium for the toxins to be flushed out of the body.

Remember that when your body has the tools it needs to work with then it will always move itself towards better health. Just help your body to help itself.

Superfoods that Fight Chronic Fatigue
Syndrome

Healing the Villi

Once your body is cleansed of toxins, it can at last begin to absorb nutrients properly once again. As we discussed earlier, most nutrient absorption occurs in the villi of the small intestine. The small intestine is about 22 feet (7 meters) long and is coiled inside the abdomen.

Within the internal walls of that long tube are villi, tiny little projections that stick out like a carpet of fine fingers, pointed toward the center.

Upon the surface of these villi are yet another surface layer of even finer micro-villi which are even more delicate but which dramatically increase the overall surface area of your villi.

Studies have indicated that the total 'surface area' of the small intestine in a healthy male can be around the area of 2 soccer ovals!

As the liquefied food passes through the intestine, these villi projections absorb the nutrition and carry them to the bloodstream.

When these villi aren't healthy, the body's ability to absorb nutrients is impaired. That ideal surface area of 2 soccer ovals can be reduced to as little as the area of a tennis court!

If that happens then you can eat as many wonderful organic super foods as you can and you still will not get the full nutritional benefits. It is critical to absorbing of nutrition to protect the health of your villi.

Many people are walking around with villi that are damaged, brittle, and broken. You may not have realized it, but there are many things that can actually cause distress to the small intestine.

First and foremost, a poor diet is a terrible thing for the small intestine. This means a diet high in saturated fat, refined sugars, chemically processed foods, and low in fiber.

Unfortunately, this describes the average diet of someone living in an industrialized country.

Food allergies also cause inflammation. For example, with celiac disease a gluten allergy begins an autoimmune response in the body. This directly attacks the villi of the small intestine leaving them inflamed and potentially diseased.

Eating at irregular times of the day is also a problem for your villi. Many people eat one big meal a day and nothing else the rest of the day. The body is really made to be fueled with small meals that take place many times throughout the day.

Superfoods that Fight Chronic Fatigue Syndrome

Not getting enough sleep or sleeping during the day can also lead to problems with the small intestine. Sleep is the time when you seem to be doing nothing, but it's actually a busy time for the body as it repairs cells and produces new ones. This can be a particular problem for shift workers.

Environmental toxins are also like poison for the villi that can cause them to become brittle and break. Instead of being soft and supple, if they become brittle then they're unable to do their job properly.

Another big factor for health of your villi is the stress in your life. A stressful lifestyle can also be very damaging for your whole body and particularly for the walls of the small intestine. If you're like most people in today's world, you're undergoing your fair share of stress.

And finally, antibiotics can cause damage to the intestines and if you are already pushing yourself, working too hard, getting too little or irregular sleep, not eating well and/or under stress in your lifestyle then antibiotics can be a huge factor in your wellness.

The body has a fine balance of good bacteria that keep the gut healthy. While antibiotics kill off the bad bacteria, they have the added effect of killing off the good bacteria. That leaves the gut stripped of these helpers that make digestion move more smoothly. This often leads to energetically impaired villi.

And even if you don't take prescription antibiotics, it's possible to be exposed to them from the food you eat. Especially when it comes to animal products, antibiotics are well known to make their way into the food supply.

Villi that are in bad shape can lead to problems such as feeling low energy levels and sleep that isn't restful. Incidentally, these are the same symptoms someone with Chronic Fatigue Syndrome experiences.

Having unhealthy villi means that, in spite of your efforts to eat healthy foods, you're not absorbing the nutrition from them and your body is actually in a state of starvation.

Healthy villi lead to higher energy levels, better rest, and better health.

Once your body is initially detoxed and cleared of toxins, it's important to restore the health of the villi in the small intestine. Herbal based natural nutritional products have herbs that are specifically designed to help the villi regenerate and become healthy once again.

The really good news is that once you begin adding the Herbal supplements to your diet, you'll begin to feel reenergized in a matter of a few short days. It won't take long before you realize that you've got more energy than you've had in quite a while.

Absorbing Nutrients

Finally, once the body has been cleared of toxins and the villi are regenerated, you'll be free to absorb the nutrients that you put into your body. The villi will be able to take in nutrients through their large surface area.

Those nutrients will be transported to the bloodstream and lymph system where they can be delivered to the appropriate structures in the body.

Rather than experiencing vitamin deficiency, you'll feel energized by the foods you eat and the vitamins in the supplements.

For you, the benefits include:

More energy
Better sleep (waking up refreshed rather than waking up and still feeling tired)
Improved immunity
Lower risk for illnesses such as diabetes and cancer
Decreased symptoms from Chronic Fatigue Syndrome

Once people experience proper nutrition, they often report feeling better than they ever have before in their lives.

And this effect is a result of just a few days using top quality nutritional supplement products that help your body to become detoxified, repaired, and open to nutrients.

Athletes and people in peak fitness sometimes feel the effect of such supplementation within a few hours. Normal, healthy, people generally feel an energy shift in about 3 days.

People with seriously energetically impaired villi and low metabolic rate can take 7 to 10 days to feel that shift.

People with serious health issues or serious CFS can take anywhere from a week to up to 6 weeks to begin to feel their health turning around and begin improving.

The time frames of how long it will take an individual to feel different are dependent upon the initial health situation of the individual involved.

The Body Heals Itself

When you take a prescription medication, it generally takes over the natural processes of the body and works to create an artificial mechanism to stop symptoms or to eradicate disease.

After the medication course is finished, you may be free from a bacterial infection or viral infection, but your body isn't any more able to heal you than it was before the medication was introduced.

However, with the application of herbal based natural nutritional supplements your body is still the one in charge. The supplement is a tool that allows your body to get back to doing its job properly. It actually heals itself.

While the supplements facilitate the process of removing toxins and restoring villi to their natural state, the true benefits that come from true nutrition are ones that your body can achieved for itself with a healthy digestive system.

If you have Chronic Fatigue Syndrome, in all likelihood your body is suffering right now from poor nutrition. You may have thought you were doing everything correctly by eating many fruits and vegetables, keeping your protein up, or lowering the fat in your diet.

But even if you improve your diet significantly, it's hard for the body to take in those nutrients correctly. And because food isn't as packed with nutrients as it once was, it may not be enough.

Natural herbal based supplements will support your body's natural healing process and help to make up for the lack of nutrients in the foods you eat. But, that doesn't mean that you can throw out the principles of a healthy diet.

Working Hand in Hand

While we have all kinds of science and technology that allows us to produce drugs to fight disease, it's becoming more and more evident that the true medication that will heal is nutritious food and regular exercise.

Many people look at food as medicine. Changing your diet and making sure you take in the important nutrients every day can help improve just about every health condition. Eliminating as many artificial ingredients as possible will benefit your body immensely.

Supplements can be used to support the body so that the nutrients you eat can be properly absorbed. They can also fill in the holes when your food doesn't provide enough of the good stuff you need.

Working together, supplements and a healthy diet can provide you with the healing you've been seeking. It's not a magic "cure" for your Chronic Fatigue Syndrome. However, the improvements you'll see in energy levels and sleep patterns will prove to you that healing is happening.

Superfoods that Fight Chronic Fatigue Syndrome

In the next section you'll learn more specific information about the kinds of supplements and nutritional products that are available on the market and how you can use them to achieve optimum health. You'll find this complementary therapy is worth your time and attention.

Chapter Five:
Supplements For A Healthy Villi
How Using Herbal Supplements Helps Turn Around CFS

Before we talk about specific nutritional supplements we want to have a more broad-brush look at the whole subject of using supplements and of keeping your body healthy. Regardless of which nutrition products you use there are some basics that you should already aware of but which we want to go over again now anyway as they are so critical to your overall health.

This is talking about things like choosing the right nutrition program in the first place, one that suits your personal situation, and then allowing *time* for healing to happen, rather than expecting instant results. The water we should all be drinking every day is another factor as is detoxification and its effects whether that comes from cleaning herbs or any other detox program.

These are foundation areas of information that you are most likely very familiar with but it is better to talk about them again here than risk you not having full information on them.

The very first step of course is that you need to consider what the best thing is for *you* in *your* specific situation before you begin on any program for healing. It's very easy to read up on nutrition and get one person's view which says a specific herb, or a specific vitamin or mineral, or a specific diet, may be the answer for your health problem.

Often such opinions suggest that theirs is the 'only' answer and that one specific action or supplement will solve everything. Instead, we should look at this in with a much broader context.

Talking with doctors and with medical professionals they often tell us that the best way to deal with Chronic Fatigue Syndrome is for the sufferer to put themselves into a 'stress free' environment, eat good nutritious meals 3 times a day, get regular sleep of at least 8 hours a night, and over 12 months or so they will recover from it.

Now many of us would have some serious reservations about this being a realistic solution for our own case and our lifestyles, but if you stop for a while and think it through, the underlying concepts are very solid.

We will talk more about 'stress' as a critical factor in CFS later. For now it is worth just considering the medical response of not treating the condition but of putting the patient into a stress free and supportive *environment* and allowing the body to heal itself over 12 months.

The key here is that your body has a God given ability to function well and to deal with the things that you throw at it.

Start walking a few minutes every single day and you will get fitter. Build up to jogging and doing sets of sprints every day and you will get even fitter still, and will probably also lose weight and reshape.

Work with heavy weights in a gym every day and you will build muscle. This tells us that when we put our bodies under stress the body will work to deal with the new conditions and adjust itself to be able to handle the new demands it faces.

This process of our body function also applies directly to wellness and to sickness. If we take away the factors that are contributing to the problem (like stress), and give the body the tools it needs to heal itself, it will always move itself towards wellness.

In our experience, with the right nutrition products this healing process can happen in a matter of weeks, not months. How to help get that happing for you is the core of what this book is about.

We are going to also look closely at the practical 'how to' methods of using supplements to beat chronic fatigue syndrome. But there is a lot more to it than just describing the methods of taking products or the quantities to take.

Initially you need to get your head around how your digestive system works, and how it becomes energetically compromised to the point where your body can't absorb the nutrition you feed it, no matter how high quality.

We are talking about helping to remove the factors that are contributing to your CFS in the first place. Then once we have your system cleared of toxins and better able to absorb nutrition through properly functioning villi, and you are giving it broad, high quality nutrition, then at last your body has the tools it needs to heal itself.

We are talking about wellness here rather than dealing with sickness.

This is something we've touched on already but it's worth focusing attention on it in a bit more detail here just so we have the same understanding of where a focused nutrition program fits into your health program.

Often people who have a CFS condition say that they have tried everything they can find to achieve wellness and, because of that, they are understandably skeptical. To take on something else requires having enough information to have confidence in what they are doing.

Confidence is something that we believe is critical for you to be successful when you embark on something new with CFS. Nutritional therapies, like many alternative therapies need to be applied with common sense and the help of experts in the field.

And this is not a battle between prescribed therapies from your doctor versus natural therapies. We're not saying here that we should separate ourselves from the health professionals like doctors and that you should not talk with them. Medical professionals are an integral part of a rounded health strategy.

If you break an arm you go to a doctor and get it set. If you have a bad infection then you get it diagnosed and get a prescription to use antibiotics. Doctors and the medical profession are critical to our society.

Superfoods that Fight Chronic Fatigue Syndrome

The medical professions normally only deal with sickness and while very professional about how they work in that area, when it comes to lifestyle factors and nutrition and diet and dealing with stress and environmental factors, we sometimes need to look for alternate answers to the limited treatments they offer.

There is a perception that 'Alternate Medicine' is opposed to 'Traditional Medicine'.

But it is preferable to see the two areas as being different parts of the same jigsaw puzzle as you try to piece together a picture of optimum health for yourself

Despite assorted media reports to the contrary we are not seeing any proof that diet and herbal nutrition will cure cancer. There is no 'magic cure' here.

But many renowned doctors have stated that that 70% of morbidity and mortality (sickness and death) have diet related causes. Also quoted was that up to 80% of bowel cancer could be avoided with inclusion of higher levels of fiber in the diet and regular exercise.

This is mentioned not so much to focus on those specific numbers but to highlight that lifestyle and nutrition are critical factors that underpin our health and that are very often contributory factors to sickness and specific medical conditions.

The issue with CFS is that it can be expressed better for many people as a 'lack of wellness' instead of being as a specific illness.

For the last few decades diagnosis of CFS has involved a process of excluding, one by one, every know illness that could cause the symptoms that the CFS patient exhibits. When it has been shown that none of those other conditions are the cause then the diagnosis of CFS can be applied.

Nowadays there are blood tests used that may show certain indicators that the problem is CFS but, frankly, this is still a very imprecise process.

If we are not dealing with a clearly defined medical condition then it is difficult for medical professionals to provide an answer. No specific condition means no specific medications that can be prescribed to deal with it.

When it comes to 'wellness', and being well, as opposed to dealing with sickness, then we have to go back to basics. We need to remove the factors that contribute to the problem and to give your body the tools it needs to heal itself.

Superfoods that Fight Chronic Fatigue Syndrome

We will cover this in more detail later and look at the process of detoxification and rebuilding of your body's ability to absorb nutrition and then giving your body high quality, broad spectrum, nutrition so that it can use those tools to heal itself.

We do that personally in our lives, and for the people we work with, by using high quality herbal based nutrition supplements in our healing.

It makes sense that a foundation of using nutrition supplements should not be to 'Cherry Pick' one supplement here, one vitamin there, in an attempt to try and to prescribe a "CFS cure".

The key is to get the best quality nutrition supplementation you can, in a herbal base to promote detoxification, and then to give the body a broad spectrum of everything your body needs so that it can work towards bringing you to better health.

Based on this, when it comes to selecting and starting to use supplements:

Don't go to the bulk discount warehouse and buy cheap supplements and think that you are getting better value.

Don't try to 'target' specific issues with specific herbs and minerals.

Do give your body all of the tools it needs to detoxify itself, and allow it to move towards wellness on as many levels as you can.

This leads us to working out the process of choosing supplements that will achieve the outcomes we are looking for.

How Do You Choose The Most Suitable Supplements?

First of all, find someone who knows what they are talking about based on their having practical experience with the nutritional supplementation products they use.

In the case of Warren Tattersall, hehas personally been working with nutrition supplements for over 20 years and has over time developed personal and professional preferences about what products are best in his experience.

In his own words Warren will now present the information on how he uses nutritional supplementation to help others beat CFS:

In my opinion, over twenty years of experience with helping people overcome health issues like CFS means that I know what I am talking about with the products that I use. But that also means that my opinion is predisposed to lean in that direction and so you will need to judge what I say here, knowing that this bias will apply to my view and my recommendations.

As I am talking about specific use of products and health outcomes we cannot name any specific products or brand names. They are food products and therefore are legally are restricted from making any 'health claims' or therapeutic claims for them.

People working with nutrition supplements are generally not medical professionals and so cannot talk about supplements actually 'curing' anything and cannot make medical claims for a product.

Often nutritional supplements have not been through full clinical trials and so any benefits that people generally gain from them cannot be guaranteed to happen for all people so again, formal claims cannot be made about health benefits of the products.

For this reason I'm not going to talk about any specific brand but instead I will discuss the most common core nutritional properties of certain products available on the market and about how to use supplements generally for your wellbeing.

If you wish to contact me for more information about what products I prefer to work with myself then you can send an email to the address at the end of this book in the About the Authors section and I will be happy to talk about these things in a personal consultation with you in more depth.

In general, when you are talking with anyone else in the field of nutritional consultants, check the background of the person giving the information and be wary, even a little skeptical, about the personal bias they bring with them. Anyone who has an opinion that is not based upon personal experience and from working directly with people who have had CFS should be treated with caution in my opinion.

So, now that I have formally declared my own personal interest and bias toward the specific products I use myself and recommend to others, we can move on to the practicalities of how to use natural nutritional supplements generally in your diet to beat CFS!

If you have studied foods in any depth then you will be aware of the difference in nutritional value between raw foods and cooked foods, organic grown food and many commercially grown crops, products that have been in long term cold store and products that are fresh from the field.

The same sort of differences apply to herbal supplements and to vitamins sourced from a natural source as opposed to chemically derived supplements

Superfoods that Fight Chronic Fatigue Syndrome

Quality Herbal nutrition products are normally sold with a money back guarantee that says if they do not work for you as you expect them to then you can return them within the first 30 days for a full refund. You should also have a nutritional consultant available to you who will talk with you and guide you on the specific use of the products and to support you as you are using them.

When you choose a nutrition supplement to assist you with CFS you really need something that is closer to quality foods than it is to a pharmaceutical product.

I suggest that you keep the concept of 'broad spectrum nutrition' in the front of your mind also.

Shortly I will cover the specific style of products that I believe are most effective but first there is some more general information that we need to cover which applies to any supplement you decide to use to ensure you get the full benefit of them.

Take Supplements Consistently

When you have nutrition products in hand, particularly herbal products, you need to take them on a regular pattern. To pull the poisons that have built up in your system out your body you use cleansing herbs.

Herbs are a plant product and they get into your system quickly but they also get out quickly. To keep active herbs in your body you need to be replacing them about every 8 hours.

Now, in reality, this would be a pain to try and maintain so the recommended process is to take herbal supplements when you would normally eat, or with your normal meals, 3 times a day.

Mostly they can be taken with your food or if you are using nutrition 'shake' as a meal replacement, then with the shake.

Give It Time to Work in Your System.

If you are using supplements properly you will not be trying to deal with symptoms, but with the underlying problem.

If you have a pain and you use a painkiller then the pain goes away. Great. Well, it *would* be great if your body was actually *dealing* with the problem and the pain was going to go anyway because the problem was cured.

Actually the use of pain killers just makes the problem less painful. If the painkillers are 'masking' the problem and not fixing it then maybe it is not so great. That is a way that can potentially lead to much bigger problems in the future.

With Herbs and nutritional supplements you are trying to deal with the underlying problems and are not seeking instant outcomes. You need to allow 'time' to be a factor in your healing.

You would not normally take a supplement and get the outcome you want in 20 minutes.

On the other hand you do need to see measurable progress in measurable time.

If you take the supplements for 90 days and have not seen any change then continuing to do the same thing in the same way and expecting a different outcome may be a problem.

If you are not getting a measurable outcome in a reasonable time then you should go back to the drawing board and start looking for alternate solutions.

The nutrition products I work with have a guarantee about the customer being happy with their health progress within the first 30 days, and if someone is not happy then they can cancel their product use, return the unused portion, and receive a 100% money back refund.

For many people who provide supplements they may not have the resources to offer that but I mention it as an indicator that within the first 30 days most people *Should* be seeing *Some* measurable outcomes from the supplements that you use.

The only time that this may not be the case is where people have CFS from an underlying chemical contamination. If your body is full of damaging chemicals and you are using supplements to leech those chemicals out they you are likely to initially feel worse rather than better during the first 30 days.

Some outcome *may* mean challenges as you clear the toxins and chemicals and then beginning to feel much better will follow. Provided you do things gently, and I will tell you exactly how to do that shortly, you should not have a bad reaction.

The outcome that we do not want to see is for there to be no change. If you are doing things properly there should be some measurable change that you can feel for yourself within the first 30 days.

When working with nutrition products, even if you start feeling better in the first month, you should then set your focus on using something for 90 days to establish solid positive results.

Just make sure you think in terms of a week at a time rather than watching the minute hand on your watch to measure the results.

Drink Enough Water

When you use cleansing herbs you should expect to detoxify chemicals and poisons and general gunk from your system. Most of that will end up in your bloodstream. You can be carrying a toxin load in your blood many times higher than normal and that can lead to the signs of Detoxification. I will cover that in a moment but first let's talk about the solution.

The solution to having such a load of toxins in your blood stream is to drink enough water to allow your body to flush them out through your kidneys and urine.

Traditional advice is that you should be drinking 2 litres/ 2 quarts of water a day, that can be taken as a rough guide as 8 large glasses of water.

I have seen writings that say you can use too much water and some to say that 2 lt is not enough so and various opinions that appear authoritive seem to contradict each other.

Because of this I recently did some research on the scientific material that has originated from studies into water use. I will not go into that in depth here but the summary of that research from the top medical sources in the world is basically that the recommended water use should be around 1 lt/quart of water per every 25 kg/55 lb of body weight.

I am 185cm/6 ft 2 in and get into a gym a bit so for me that is saying that 4 Lt/qt is more in line with what I should be using.

This research was to understand what I *Should* be doing myself and I admit that my water use is well below 4 litres a day. From checking this though it is clear that using 2 lt/qt a day is a realistic minimum water use for most people.

When changing your diet and adding supplements then if you are suffering any signs of detoxification then you can feel pretty comfortable in increasing the volumes of water you are drinking to help flush through your system and know that you are not drinking too much water.

When you are counting your water remember that tea and coffee are diuretics. That means they draw water Out Of your body. You cannot count tea or coffee into your water intake for the day or, if you do count them, you should actually count them as negative to your daily total.

Replacing Tea and Coffee with water gives a double effect of reducing the diuretic effect of the drink actually taking water out of your system and gives the positive effect of adding in the water you actually drink. It is a bit of a challenge for many of us to make that shift but if you even take some of the diuretic drinks you have in a normal day and replace them with water you will be doing your body a favour.

If you do not drink much water then adding enough water into your day it hard but it is worth doing.

At the *Very Least* it is important that you pay particular attention to this in the first 2 or 3 weeks of a detox program when it is most critical to have high water use as there is much more toxin to be flushed out of your system than normally.

What is Detox?

In the last few pages we talked about use of water and how important it is. Here I would like to run over that mystical Detox issue.

When people talk about Detox they are talking about doing something to assist their body to remove the toxins from their body. Removing toxins, detoxifying, detox, they are different words that say the same thing.

How do we get the toxins into our system in the first place?

Build-up of waste products your own body produces.

Poisons you breathe in just from the air you breathe – this can be significant in rural areas where there are air born chemicals from farming in addition to day to day contaminants but if you live in a city where the poisons are so thick that you can actually see them (smog) then really do have to ponder what it is doing to your body.

Environmental poisons you take in from cleaning agents, chemical solutions that get on to your skin, even from skin contact with plastics and other man made materials.

Chemicals in the food we eat from preservatives, colouring and flavouring agents through to pesticides, and hormones and growth agents introduced into the meats and the vegetables themselves as they grow.

In other words, if you live in a modern environment you will absorb poisons from your environment regardless of how careful you are.

If you live outside the cities you do avoid the smog etc but, unfortunately, it appears that rural settings have a higher incidence of CFS than cities. In my experience farming areas that are surrounded by higher land and where the air sits seem to be worst of all. People think that this us due to farm chemicals in the air.

Whatever the cause, modern living means that you need to be aware of chemicals in your system and detoxifying them occasionally is a good idea.

Detoxification Symptoms

Once you start the process of putting cleansing herbs into your system and trigger a detox process then your daily water use becomes much more important.

If you do not drink enough water and flush out those poisons with your urine then they build up in your blood stream and you can exhibit the symptoms of detox.

What are they?

These things are fairly common signs of detox:

A dull headache. That is often compared to a mild hangover if you are familiar with that feeling (A sharp headache is not likely to be associated with detox).
Muscle stiffness, a bit like if you have done a workout and have tired muscles. This is typically in the shoulders, neck, upper back and also lower back around the kidneys.

Maybe light headedness
Bad breath.
Smelly feces.

People with skin blemishes, pimples for example, can find that they will get worse as your body pushes the poisons out through the skin before they get better. Take heart though if this happens, as in my experience people who experience this have often had a long term problem and if they go through a bad period in clearing this sort of problem it is normal to finish that and have the skin become better and clearer than it has been for a very long time, often better than it has ever been.

Worse than normal body odour.

Anything else that involves a process for your body to push toxins out is likely to be related to your detoxification.

Some of these symptoms seem unpleasant and you would want them to stop. There are 2 ways you get rid of these symptoms:

The first is to stop doing the activity that is causing the detox. That can mean to stop taking the herbal supplements, get off the raw food diet, stop blending healthy juices and adding them to your diet. If you stop your body clearing these poisons into your blood stream then you will stop the symptoms of a high toxin load trying to leave your body.

The second option is to keep doing what you are doing, clearing out the poisons, and to increase the water you are drinking so your body can flush out the poisons as the water flushes through your system.

It just seems logical that if you can clean your body in the same simpler manner that you clean your car or clean up dishes then you should do it. Your body will be with you a lot longer than your car and if it gets old and stops working efficiently you cannot trade it in for a new one.

If you think about any potential discomfort with having to drink extra water for cleansing then also think at the same time how you want to be feeling in the last 20 years of your life. For a healthy and happy old age you need to do some things now so you will keep well.

The other thing that I always have in the back of my mind is that I keep hearing about medical studies looking into links between environmental toxins in your body and developing cancer, there are hundreds of studies going on around the world.

Personally I don't want to wait another 10 years for those studies to prove out the theories and then find I should have done something about dealing with pollution and environmental toxins 10 years earlier. Better to do it now and not take that risk.

The Side Effects of a 'Change of Diet' Can Derail Your New CFS Diet.

I am trying to prepare you to succeed with your activity to get healthy by showing you the potential traps and pitfalls on your path. If you know what they are then it is not hard to avoid them or, if you have a problem, you know what it is and so know how to deal with it.

Another issue when you change your eating program is the very 'Change of Diet'.

This is just what it says; if you change the diet you are eating then your body may react to that change.

If you smoke and then one day you stop you can expect withdrawal symptoms. They can be very hard, painful, even debilitating.

If you drink 6 large beers after work every night then it may well be a cause of weight gain. If you decide to do something about that and just stop drinking one day, cold turkey, it is probably going to give you withdrawal problems.

Superfoods that Fight Chronic Fatigue Syndrome

Coffee is endemic in our society and has become part of the culture. Many people have a strong coffee to start the day and more coffee during the day. May people top it up with sugar.

If you are having 4 or 5 coffees during the day then if you stop, cold turkey, and suddenly change to drinking no coffee at all you can expect to have change of diet issues.

Coffee is a diuretic. That means that it draws liquids out of your body. Estimates vary depending on the scientific source you listen to but it seems fair to say that if you drink one strong cup of coffee then the fluid from that will pass through your system and also take with it ½ to 1 cup of water out of your system.

Studies are showing that taking a tea bag and making a cup of tea can have similar diuretic effects as a cup of coffee so if you are a tea drinker it may be worth investigating herbal teas.

If you stop drinking coffee suddenly and your body does not have a chance to adjust then you will not have that extra liquid in your bowel and you can expect to become constipated, maybe even badly constipated.

You are likely to get sharp headaches from caffeine withdrawal.

You are likely to become tense and irritated, again from caffeine withdrawal.

These are classic 'Change Of Diet' symptoms. If you reduce the coffee intake slowly over a period of time you would expect to not have these side effects.

If you have high sugar levels in your diet and you stop them overnight then your body will react. I imagine that you are aware that many commercial drinks: soft drink, flavoured milk, even commercial fruit juices can have up to 12 spoons of sugar per can/bottle.

If you have a can of soft drink with lunch and another with dinner then you are talking around 24 spoons of sugar just there. Doing that means you have no right to criticize work colleagues who put 3 or 4 spoons of sugar in their coffee, they are having a lot less sugar than you are!

It also means that if you stop it overnight your body is likely to react to the change so you need to be aware of it.

If you have high fat levels in your diet and you stop them overnight then your body will react.

If you have high salt levels in your diet and you stop them overnight then your body will react.

Most processed and packed food in our modern society are packed full of sugar, fats and salt.

81

Superfoods that Fight Chronic Fatigue Syndrome

Why am I making such an issue of this?

If you find the right supplements, choose a raw food diet, do something to get yourself healthy, and begin that while cutting out everything bad in your diet and *You Don't Drink Enough Water* then you may have detox symptoms and 'Change of Diet' symptoms all at the same time.

I have heard people say: *"I went on that diet and it almost killed me. I had headaches, muscles were sore, dizziness, stomachaches. I thought I was going to die. As soon as I stopped it I felt better again"*.

When I talk with those people they were normally not aware of keeping their water up and they cut out a heap of things from their diet overnight. When they reintroduced the cigarettes, the fats, the sugar, the caffeine then they stabilized, their bodies stopped clearing the poisons out of their system and the symptoms disappeared.

This is why I'm going through these things in detail for you. I believe myself that if you leave the poisons in your muscles and in your vital organs it may not mean too much to you now but over time it is like leaving things outside in the weather, there will be long term damage, and when you are old and should be enjoying travel and family and having time for your hobbies you may not have the health to do it.

The cost of missing out on those things far outweighs the cost of doing something about it now while you can.

Before moving on I need to give some practical answers to dealing with Change of Diet.

The first and most important thing you have already done. It is getting some information on what you are dealing with and understanding it. The fact that you are reading this puts you further ahead of the general population than I can tell you.

Most people, and I do mean most people, decide they need to do something for their health, take advice from friends or family or popular magazines and just go ahead and do it. They do not study, they do not read and they do not ponder what they are trying to achieve. You are doing all of these things and I congratulate you.

To deal with Change of Diet the key is to not cut things out - but to just cut back instead.

If you finish work and have 6 beers then when you finish your work try having 2 beers. You will find you actually enjoy them more and it will give your body a chance to adjust.

You may even start going 6 to 4 for a few days or a week and then down to 2 for a while. You may stay on 2 or cut them out altogether but doing it progressively will mean that your body can adjust as you get yourself to where you want to be.

If you drink 8 cups of coffee a day then think about choosing 2 times in the day when you have a coffee and stick to just those 2. It will reduce the effects of the dietary change.

If you are going towards a full raw food diet then you will probably want to get the coffee out of your diet all together but I strongly recommend that you do that in stages and withdraw the coffee, the soft drink, the high fat foods gradually and not just overnight.

You can be strong and just change if you are aware of the things you may need to deal with but personally I prefer people to step into the changes without discomfort and move towards a permanent change of habits that can stay with them for the rest of their lives.

Taking time to develop sustainable healthy eating will also allow you to take into account that food is 'social', it is a part of our whole social fabric, and learning to eat healthy while still being able to maintain social relationships is worth thinking about and putting some effort into getting right.

Here are links for more reading on these issues that you may find useful:

http://www.thehealthsuccesssite.com/change-of-diet.html

http://www.thehealthsuccesssite.com/detoxification-details-article.html

Natural Herbal Nutritional Supplementation Therapy

We who work in the nutrition industry are required to never prescribe; we do not deal in medications. Anyone competent in the alternative health area will never give advice on the medications that medical professions have prescribed or recommended for you.

Sorry to sound 'wishy washy' but if we are going to be helpful for you then we need to be very transparent with everything we say and we also ensure these 'housekeeping' things are covered.

There is not necessarily any conflict between nutrition, which would include vitamin and mineral supplementation and eating programs involving super-foods or raw food diets, on the one side and medically prescribed medication on the other.

Vitamin and mineral supplementation and eating programs are food. They need to be used wisely and everything you do with diet and how you treat your body has effects so you need to review information in depth and then make informed decisions.

Superfoods that Fight Chronic Fatigue Syndrome

You are reading this book and that indicates that you research and study things. This is the best thing you can be doing for a CFS condition initially. Once you have some clarity in understanding what it is and how you want to work with dealing with it then you have a solid foundation to build on.

Part of that research is to know what to expect when you embark on any specific course and to do it in a sensible, measured and sustainable manner.

If you are involving vitamin and mineral supplements you have guidelines of how much of anyone ingredient is healthy and I recommend that you understand and respect those guidelines.

In this book I am not going to be recommending that you use Mega-Doses of any particular ingredient.

I will also never give medical advice or make medical claims for nutritional products.

That means that I ask you to think of the foods we talk about as food and also that you think of food supplements as food.

Good quality supplements that are not derived from chemical sources and that involve quality herbs and botanical factors can be thought of as leaves, twigs and berries that are chopped and crushed, blended with the vitamins, and pressed together in tablet form so that you can get the right amount of each ingredient in the right balance every time.

Eating that sort of supplement is like eating fruit. Can you eat an apple? Yes? Then you can use nutrition supplements in accordance with the labeling on the bottles.

There are 2 factors that go into the labeling that I want to mention here:

The first is the mega-dose laws that if there is too much of any one ingredient in a product then it cannot be sold

The second is that if anything in such a product can affect an individual then it must be stated on the label. – This is why you see aspirin based products with warnings not to use them when using heavy equipment as there is a risk of drowsiness for some people. You see some products with warnings that they are not recommended for pregnant or lactating (breast feeding) women.

These things mean that if you are using a commercial product that has been approved for sale in a developed country, like USA for example, then these tests and standards will have been applied.

In other words, used as described on the label they may not be able to guarantee that the products will be good for you but we do know that the products will not do you any harm.

Beside that we have drugs and medications that can be very powerful and effective tools for your health but that can also be very dangerous and that can be contraindicated to other medications and mixing them can be dangerous.

The risks here are so great that these drugs and medications are severely restricted in how they are sold. Medical doctors spend years studying so they have the skill set needed to be able to understand what is available and so they can legally prescribe them for you.

The pharmacist who gives you the products spends years studying so they can understand what they are giving you and not give you medications that you will take in the wrong dose or that will react badly with each other.

Just by the way, if a doctor accidentally prescribes a medication at 10 times the correct strength and the pharmacist supplies that medication to you and it harms or kills you then it is the pharmacist who is ultimately responsible as they are the official backup to ensure that medications issued are all within safe dosages.

When you think in these terms you see that these two worlds of natural healing and medical intervention are very different. They are both working towards your better health though so they overlap each other. This can sometimes cause confusion as people are torn between one and the other.

It is important that we take this short time to review that and to understand how they fit together.

Natural health practitioners cannot make health claims. They can tell you what has happened for other people and that naturally lets you think "Well if it worked for them and I have a similar situation tem maybe it will work for me".

Natural healing involves you taking a strong measure of personal responsibility and doing the research and study, pondering, and then putting together the things that you believe will move you towards better health. Natural healing will give you information and options but you need to assess them for yourself and use them wisely.

You may find that is seems obvious to you and you may decide to change the way you use medication or discontinue using them. The correct way to do that is to do so in conjunction with your doctor.

You may go to them and say that you want to try some alternate methods and will they monitor your progress for you. You may ask if there is any short term risk in ceasing using a medication. Doctors with a broad experience will normally support you in this.

Others may believe that medications are the only answer and not support you but my main point here is that this is between you and your doctor and no-one outside has any right to interfere with anything the doctor is doing.

When it comes to supplements they are a food product. The mega-dose laws and the labeling laws are in place to cover you. If a product was contra-indicated to a medication then it needs to be listed on the label. If you want to get an opinion from your doctor on using supplements then I recommend that you do so.

There is a way to talk this through with you doctor that will give you a clear answer and that is also fair to your doctor. In years of study for a medical degree there are only a handful of hours dedicated to nutrition and you cannot expect a General Practitioner to be an expert on nutrition supplements.

Since the American Medical Association indicates that around 70% of sickness and death is based in nutritional causes the lack of time doctors spend studying nutrition seems completely out of balance but that is the medical profession directing what is studied, not your doctor.

If you ask for his/her opinion about whether a specific supplement will do you any good they are professionally bound by their answer. It is moving outside what they have studied and what they have worked with and it goes against the interests of the drug companies so there have been many negative opinions given to the doctor.

If you ask if a supplement that the doctor is not supplying will be good for you then you are unlikely to get a positive answer.

The best way to approach a doctor is to take a bottle of the supplement, or a copy of the label, to them and ask this question:

"Doctor, is there anything in this that could do me any *harm*?"

Now you have a question that the doctor is free to answer as the labeling law and the mega-dose law comes into play and knowing that the doctor is free to give their opinion.

You can expect a response that varies on one end of the response scale from your doctor saying that they really don't know if such products will do you any good, even that they doubt they will do you any good, but that there is nothing in them that will do you any harm, to the other end where they will be interested and supportive of you working with alternate health options.

Nowadays many doctors are looking at nutrition and lifestyle factors in people's health and if you have a doctor that is doing that they will probably be happy to monitor your progress as you use alternate, non-medical, methods to improve your health and wish to keep an eye on your progress.

Even so, there are still some doctors who are very negative about anything that does not originate from the drug companies. In that case you have to make your own decision about if you continue to take that doctor's advice.

It is very important to us as I have said though that you make your own decision about working with medical professionals and in this book you will not find anything giving advice on medications or interfering with your current relationship with your doctor.

Now we are nearly to the point of discussing the actual kinds of nutritional supplements to use in conjunction with key superfoods, but first you need to learn how to evaluate what level of CFS stage you are going to have to deal with and recognize what your triggers or causes may be.

This is because your degree or depth of chronic fatigue syndrome requires different methods of easing into and ratios of supplement product use.

Discovering Your Own Level of CFS and Your Triggers

Chronic Fatigue Syndrome is a difficult thing to define as all the information has shown.

At the start of this book you saw the official summary of CFS signs and symptoms as recognized by most medical practitioners, but they are not really comprehensive enough in my opinion.

What I find normally when talking with people is that there seems to be several histories that are common to people with Chronic Fatigue Syndrome.

I'd like to go through those with you now so you can see these backgrounds to align with your own and you can see if you find a reflection of yourself in here.

In my experience of working with CFS sufferers I have seen that:

Many will have had a high, or elevated, stress period in their lives and during that time they will have had a health "incident". In most cases that will have involved the use of antibiotics. Some time after that, normally 3 to 6 months, they noticed that they were tired most of the time and little problems with their health started to become apparent. This often includes sports people.

Separately, but still falling into the same stress/incident category, are people who have had a viral infection that appeared to clear up but that they never felt they recovered completely. They then slipped into a downhill path that has left them with the conditions of Chronic Fatigue Syndrome.

Next there is a group who has had chemical contamination and this is the group that is most difficult to draw back from the edge of immune system collapse. Sometimes these individuals can look back at their lives and identify a source, often that source was a long way back in their past, even from childhood and sometimes these people have been dealing with the issues of CFS at some level for most of their lives.

People who have had major substance abuse issues. This would include people recovering from drug addiction or other major chemical issues. These people are a special case in my view as there is so much going on in dealing with the original problems and walking the long path back to better health and control of their lives the CFS symptoms just get jumbled in with the rest of the issues and are difficult to focus on.

With all of these cases there are answers and we will look at them in much more depth so that you can assess if these things are relevant to you in your own condition.

Personally I think it is important to go into these backgrounds so you can assess if your own situation compared to these and if you can select a 'category' or level. If you can do that then you find it easier to go through our section on using nutrition products to assist with your CFS.

As I have said, I do not have a medical background and I cannot give medical advice. On the other hand, if I was talking with someone who did not understand my condition then I would be hesitant to take advice from them.

If was talking with someone who could explain to me some of the history of how I got to be the way I am and who fully understood what it is like to be living with the condition then I would be a lot interested to listen to their advice.

If they also had deal with many dozens of people who have had CFS and who no longer exhibit the symptoms (notice I did not use the 'cure' word) then I would be interested to look more deeply into what they had to say and to maybe take advice from them on dealing with the condition.

Superfoods that Fight Chronic Fatigue Syndrome

Do You Recognize Your Own Symptoms of CFS?

There are medical listing of symptoms that people with CFS may be expected to suffer but by the time you have read this far into a book like this one I am sure you have seem them many times.

Rather than going over those lists again I'd like to start by looking closer at the symptoms that I commonly see in people who think they may be beginning to suffer from CFS, or who have recently acquired the problem and are trying to come to terms with it.

People with a well establish CFS condition are more than familiar with what the symptoms are because they have been living with them for a long time.

The symptoms that present in the time leading up to someone realizing that they have CFS can often be a lot more subtle than the clearly defined symptoms outlined in the medical texts.

Often it can look a bit like the individual is just getting run down and working too hard. That's one of the problems with CFS, slipping from working too hard and just really needing a holiday into a condition where extra sleep and a holidays don't help can be a gradual thing.

You may only have a nagging feeling the back of your mind that 'something is just not right' and not even be really sure that you have a problem until it is so pronounced you are overwhelmed, feeling lost, for many people suffering depression, and a feeling of isolation.

The things that indicate we may have a problem are often fairly simple things like:

When you have a full night's sleep but still wake up tired.
When you have energy/concentration drop-outs in the middle of the day.
When you start having food allergies that had not been a problem, or not apparent, before.
When you start reacting to environmental conditions that had not affected you before. This may be hay fever, asthma or just sensitivity to pollution or aerosol sprays, or even to skin care products.
When your immune system starts to drop away it seems fairly common for people who previously did not get colds and flues to find that when anyone around them sneezes they pick up the bug from it. There are indicators that your immunity is lower than it was before.

Not being able to give a clear explanation to others about the problems you are experiencing leads sufferers into a cycle of helplessness, isolation and even depression.

Superfoods that Fight Chronic Fatigue Syndrome

Someone described this as like having a black cloud creeping up on them from behind and no one understanding. In that case having a medical check that says that there is nothing medically wrong can actually sharpen the fear that there really is something fundamentally wrong.

There is a difficulty with this that it engenders a feeling of helplessness and isolation alongside the low energy from the CFS. That is a mix of emotions that can lead to depression and isolation.

If this cycle is allowed to continue then it gets harder and harder for the people in early stages of CFS to have the energy and the will to actually take positive action to try and do something about it. They often come to accept the new reality of low energy, health issues, isolation and sometimes just a feeling of helplessness, even hopelessness.

I cover this so that if you are at that situation you know that we understand what you are going through. Now it is time to talk about how you got that way and what you can do to turn it all around again

What Caused Your Chronic Fatigue Syndrome?

Building on the comments before about the things that seem to be common in the history of people with CFS I will go into that in more detail so you can see which is closest to your own condition and know what to expect as you begin to deal with it.

When I sit with someone to talk about their condition with CFS and to advise how I think, in my opinion, they should use nutrition products I generally ask them how they fell and encourage them to talk through all the health and lifestyle issues they are experiencing.

What I am doing is trying to assess which of the levels above best describes their own situation.

Bear in mind that CFS is not, I believe, a specific medical condition and that everyone experiences it in different ways. We do not diagnose anything but look at the broad range of conditions to get an overview of what we are dealing with in any specific case.

Most people who have had a CFS condition for some time are pretty aware of their situation as they have had to put management practices into their daily life to be able to keep going.

When talking with people I ask them if they can identify when they first realised that they had a problem.

Most people are able to identify a specific period when they found the condition beginning to manifest.

Superfoods that Fight Chronic Fatigue Syndrome

If they can identify when the symptoms began to appear then I ask them to think back before they noticed the problem and about 6 or 8 months before, why were they using antibiotics?

Some people think that is a bit strange and some people can easily say that they had a broken arm or that they had an operation or that they had an infection of something else that caused them to be using antibiotics.

Others cannot remember using them but as we continue chatting it is pretty common for people to say "Oh, I just realized" and go on to talk about a specific event that would indeed have caused them to use antibiotics.

We then talk about the stress factors that were in their life before the period when they began to have to deal with their own CFS.

Often there is a history of stressful work, or relationship issues, of family problems with parents or children. Often these people were carers themselves looking after someone else. They may have been in a high stress job. Students going through a high tension study time are another group that we often see with CFS issues.

If there was a period of stress and then use of antibiotics then I identify the individual in my mind as probably being in Level 1 in my own reckoning, people with Impaired Ingestion

If they did not have these specific issues in their history then I talk with them to look for viral infections: Glandular fever, encephalitis, or more localized conditions with names like 'Ross River Virus' here in Australia but that refer to viral illnesses.

These people normally have no issue identifying the time of the virus. Interestingly the viral infection can have been years, sometimes many years before, and the CFS have come on very slowly since. The time delay and the gradual onset of the condition can mean that the sufferer has made no connection themselves between the two conditions.

There can be from a number of factors leading to the problem and for the sake of clarity I will list a range of incidences that I have personally encountered:

People who have been under long term stress and worry.
People who are/were working shift work especially nurses and people whose shift changes week to week so they do not develop a solid routine.
People with broken sleep patterns, especially is their eating habits are irregular.
Elite sports people, especially after they retire from

their sport.

People who have someone close to them who has been sick for some time – especially if the current sufferer was a carer for the person with the long term illness.

People who have gone through marriage or relationship breakdown.

People who have had a sudden death in the family.

People who have been under long term work pressure.

People who have been experiencing bullying.

People who have gone through a financial or similar crisis.

Students who have been pushing themselves with extended study habits.

People living in a dysfunctional relationship that causes constant pressure.

People in a job they hate.

People who are have sick family member that has caused them to worry on an ongoing basis.

What we are talking about here are people who are living a life under stress.

This condition in itself is not enough to bring on the Chronic Fatigue Syndrome problem.

Medical trials have not been able to identify the causes of the problem because within a group of people who are under stress like this some will fall to this problem and most of the others will not. There does not seem to any consistency to it.

Clearly these life stresses alone are not enough to trigger Chronic Fatigue Syndrome.

What I have found though is that the issues of lifestyle stress are commonly in the background of virtually everyone I have ever talked with who have CFS, except for where viral infections or chemical contamination are involved.

These conditions are not uncommon in modern life though so we need to ask - *what is it that triggers the CFS for these people?*

My belief is that the underlying problem for these people lies in the inability of their body to absorb nutrition from what they are eating, (energetically impaired villi – See Chapter 4).

As you have seen in the material on nutrition and absorbing nutrition the villi are the critical point from where your body absorbs nutrition and if they are not functioning properly then whatever you are eating is not being absorbs and your body will start to starve, your metabolism will drop off, you will lose energy as your tries to conserve your energy to protect you and you will begin to exhibit the onset symptoms of CFS.

Superfoods that Fight Chronic Fatigue Syndrome

What I do nowadays when talking with people who have Chronic Fatigue Syndrome, or who are showing the symptoms of onset Chronic Fatigue Syndrome, is to ask them *when and why they took* _antibiotics_.

They often look confused and I ask them to think back to about 6 months before the symptoms became really obvious and then they can normally tell me what it is that caused them to use antibiotics.

Some people initially don't recall using antibiotics but then a few minutes later will say, "Oh yes, I forgot that ... (*this happened*) ... and I used antibiotics then."

Now antibiotics in themselves are lifesavers and for many of our health problems require the use of antibiotics. If you have infection, have an operation, have an accident with broken bones and other problems then you have no choice but to use the antibiotics.

One of the side effects through of the use of these drugs through is that they damage our digestive systems. They key is knowing how to be able to benefit from medications such as antibiotics, and at the same time be able to support and assist your body in repairing the side effects of those medications.

Next we have people who have had a problem with CFS that leads back for some time, for some people they have lived with it for as long as they can remember.

Often people in this group have more allergies and food intolerances and it is not uncommon for them to be really quite sick.

If the condition reaches back to childhood I would be thinking that there is a chemical contamination issue.

If they have worked in industry then we would be looking for chemical contamination.

The geographical areas that have highest serious CFS problems tend to be rural areas. Where there are farming areas with surrounding hills to keep chemicals in the air from dispersing then there could be a hot spot for CFS.

People think of farms being wide open spaces with good clean air but if someone is working with chemicals, especially if it is an intensive farming environment then chemical contamination is a real possibility.

Of all the groups this is the hardest one to deal with. It is going to take longer to get better and there is a good chance of having problems along the way.

The final group I want to talk about is people who have, or who are, recovering from long term use of drugs.

This can be people who have has a drug addiction or it can be people who have been on medical drugs. If the drugs have been addictive or if the drugs used have psychedelic effects then there is a potential for problems when you start detoxifying them and freeing them up with your bloodstream.

These are all common triggers that you should consider when pondering what external toxin or lifestyle even may be the cause of your case of CFS as it will help you to select the most appropriate method to ease into your CFS diet and supplements later in this book.

Next I'll describe the specific properties of the core nutritional supplements I personally use and recommend.

Specific Herbal Based Nutritional Supplements for CFS Therapy

The natural herbal based nutrition products I deal with have a wide range to choose from. There are some specific products that I recommend from that range that people dealing with CFS should use.

There are a lot of products on the market which people suggest can be used to assist CFS. I have dealt a lot of people who have tried dozens and dozens of different products and not been able to turn their problem around. The obvious conclusion from that is that while there are many products out there, most of them are not effective.

On the other hand I want to cover what sort of results you can expect if you use the right nutrition products and that creates an issue. Nutrition supplements like these are a food product and so there can be no nutritional claims made about health results from using this sort of product.

The only solution to that dilemma that I can see is to give you general indicators of the sort of products to use and not identify any specific company or brand name. You can then take this information and find products that match the descriptions I have given, or you can make direct contact with me for further information about product options available to you.

My recommended nutritional supplementation therapy revolves around four key herbal based products. As I have declared earlier, I have an interest in a particular brand that I prefer myself, and would be happy to assist you with sourcing yourself, but these kinds of nutritional products are available in a variety of forms and brands if you choose to look around online or in your local health food stores.

Superfoods that Fight Chronic Fatigue Syndrome

(If you want to have direct contact with the authors regarding specific brands of nutrition products contact details for how to contact us are at the end of the book,)

1.Amino-protein powder drink.

This is a soy based product and not milk based. Personally, I strongly recommend avoiding any milk based supplements.

The Amino Protein shake is designed to give you serious nutrition with high levels of protein and amino acids without fats and unnecessary sugars.

The base of the shake is soy based protein and not dairy. Any dairy within the shake are in such small quantities that people with lactose intolerance should not have any issue with them (though this is why we are doing a detailed 'how to use to products' section here so that you can find the best way to sample products and introduce slowly and so ensure that you do not have any intolerance issues with these products).

When you hear the word 'shake' do not think 'Milk-shake'. This program avoids the use of dairy products unless you personally wish to introduce them yourself as a medium to mix the shake into.

Initially I very strongly recommend that you do not add dairy products into your diet so mix the shake in water or with fruits and berries blended, or with soy or rice milk, or yoghurt. This section covers how to use the shake itself rather than how to mix it.

Depending what country you are in the shake comes in a container with enough powder to mix about 30 shakes.

That will be about 25g of the Amino-protein shake powder.

If you have received a scoop with your Amino-protein shake then it will be 2 scoops.

If you do not have a scoop then one scoop is equivalent to 2 flat desert spoons or one flat table spoon of powder (a desert spoon is the spoon that you would normally eat a desert or a bowl of cereal with).

For people in normal health they just start using the shake at the recommended levels.

People with serious CFS problems traditionally do not introduce anything into their diet without extreme care.

I would never recommend them to go onto full strength shakes initially.

On the other hand over 50 or more people with CFS conditions who I have worked with everyone is able to use the shakes, even when they have specific food allergies that would appear to prevent them doing so.

2. Vitamin & Minerals

The second is a **broad spectrum vitamin and mineral** tablet supplement.

This is not the usual supermarket or bulk discount house variety of multivitamin.

These are a combination of herbal based natural nutrition to ensure your daily CFS diet has the full spectrum of vitamins and minerals to help maximize your recovery and maintain your new healthy state.

3. Aloe Vera Juice

Aloe heals where it touches. If you cut or graze your hand and there is an aloe vera plant nearby you can cut the succulent leaf and rub the internal gel on the wound. The discomfort will reduce quickly and the rate of healing will normally be dramatically faster than without the use of the aloe products.

Internally it is a little more difficult to apply aloe in its natural form so you need to use a high quality Aloe Vera Juice

A quality product will be clear to look at and pleasant smelling. If you find an aloe juice that is a cloudy solution that smells and tastes poorly then you will have an extract of the full juice.

This is very good for cleansing the lower bowel and is a much cheaper product but it will not deliver the same cleansing and healing properties as a juice that is extracted from just the heart of the plant.

It also cleans through your system. It has been likened to giving your body a shower on the inside. This is a good foundation to preparing to recover from chronic fatigue syndrome though it will not generate the core healing that is required by itself.

The Aloe will also cause a very gentle detoxification to begin in the body. With chemicals and drugs this will gently leach them into the blood stream where they can be flushed out of your system.

In addition to the Aloe Vera Juice another product that will help to balance the irritable bowel problem is acidophilus.

Once you have introduced Aloe Vera and allowed that to begin the cleansing of your digestive system then, when you are comfortable, you can add the Acidophilus fiber tablet.

4. The Acidophilus Fiber Tablet

The third is a **fiber tablet** with a very gentle fiber that scrubs through the bowel without irritating any digestive problems. That product also has dormant **acidophilus**.

Superfoods that Fight Chronic Fatigue Syndrome

That is a spore variety that remains dormant until you take the tab. It then breaks down but the acidophilus does not become active till it is activated by an enzyme in the small intestine.

These two products together, Aloe and the Acidophilus fiber tablet, work to promote healing through the entire digestive tract and, in many cases, even assists in bringing irritable bowel syndrome back under control and aid in preventing "flare ups".

One note, the tablets absorb water from the bowel so if you have diarrhoea problems taking one or two tablets with only a small sip of water will help reduce the fluid in the gut.

If you have constipation problems then taking an Acidophilus fiber tablet with a full glass of water is a gentle fiber that will give the added roughage you need in your diet.

Finally, as the Acidophilus fiber tablets absorb liquids, you need to not take them at the same time as the tablet will absorb the aloe and pass it out of your system before you can get the full benefit of it. Separate the two by 20 min or half an hour.

Once you have a basic cleansing and healing process happening then you should look at adding in the nutrition products to heal your whole system.

For some people a couple of days will be enough to get things moving but if you think there a high chance of chemicals or drugs being involved then using the Aloe Vera Juice and Acidophilus fiber tablet for 5 days or even a week prior to adding the shake and multivitamins to your diet is a good idea.

The problem has taken a long time to establish and it will continue to do immense harm to your system if you do not deal with it so taking enough time to work conservatively with the healing and get it right is a very advisable

In the following information, rather than talking about any specific brands, I will refer to them as:

Amino-protein shake
Multivitamin tablet
Aloe Vera juice
Acidophilus fiber tablets

The core functions of these products for dealing with CFS are to cleanse the bowel, and rebuild the villi, so that your body can then better absorb the nutrition in the foods you eat.

Then we need to give your body pure, very high quality, nutrition that includes vitamins, minerals, herbs, protein and amino acids in a balance that works together and that your body can readily absorb and deliver directly to your cells.

113

Superfoods that Fight Chronic Fatigue
Syndrome

Doctors that I personally know say that whenever you give the body the tools it needs to heal itself if will always move itself towards wellness.

This is the real key: not to give a cure for your CFS but to give your body the tools it needs to heal itself.

What to Expect When You Begin on Nutrition Supplements.

Here we are looking at what to expect when you change your diet and when you introduce broad spectrum nutrition products into the diet of someone suffering chronic fatigue syndrome.

When someone starts on nutrition program like the one suggested here they have the basic building blocks for good health. They should not be thinking in terms of medications. They should be thinking in terms of giving their body what it needs to heal itself.

In the first few days your body will work to rebuild the villi so that it can absorb nutrition. As soon as it is able to do this, then your body will start to repair itself.

An interesting, though slightly unsavoury, sign of how things are going it to watch your urine once you are on a nutrition program.

When you put the vitamins and minerals into the diet then many of them will pass straight through your system and into the toilet. It almost seems that you can *"cut out the middle man and just throw your tablets straight into the toilet!!"*

I constantly meet people who have been on nutrition supplements for extended times, sometimes years, and they are still seeing this highly coloured urine. This means that their body is passing through the urine the vitamins and especially the minerals rather than absorbing them in their body.

With the multivitamin tablets I expect people to see this high colour urine for a couple of days, or even up to a week, but as the villi rebuilds and the body then starts to absorb these mineral the colour normally reduces and the clarity returns. This means your body is absorbing what it needs to rebuild from the cells up so you can be well and healthy again.

People with Chemical contamination, or past drug issues, have deeper problems. Part of dealing with the health challenge is to detoxify the toxins out of their system.

In that detox process they will often trigger complications from the chemicals that are being released into their bloodstream. This can cause health problems that they thought they had got under control to appear to reoccur. There is a process for working through this that needs to be followed.

Superfoods that Fight Chronic Fatigue Syndrome

As the contaminates in your system leech out into your blood steam in the process of eliminating it from your body then the load of toxins in your system will be higher than normal.

During this time it is important that you drink lots of clean water. A minimum of 2 liters (2 quarts) – 8 large glasses a day – is recommended.

If you are not drinking the water then you can have symptoms like dull headaches, muscle stiffness, clouded thinking, just generally not feeling very well.

These are good signs as it means that things are happening but you do not need to put up with them.

Dealing with chemical contamination can be tough and can, in some cases, take 60 to 90 days before the benefits are apparent but not dealing with it leaves you open to continuing problems, maybe immune system collapse and if the gamut of scientific studies that are currently being run are any indication then the contamination may be linked to incidences of cancer. Doing something about the problem is critical.

As you read on from here, this is where your earlier consideration comes into play, where you decide what level or stage of CFS you are currently at including what kind of symptoms of CFS apply to you personally and where you should begin at for your nutritional therapy.

I have put in a separate section for each of the CFS histories I have listed below. If you are clear in your own mind about what information you need then just read that section.

If you wish to read through all the sections you will find some of the information is repeated in each section and you will be able to skim over the duplicate information.

Level 1. Onset CFS

Before people realize that they have a CFS condition there is generally a history of 'slipping wellness' in their lives.

Often people find that they have gone through a time of just not feeling right:

They wake up feeling tired rather than rested.

They have energy dropouts during the afternoon. Just a difficulty with concentration and motivation levels at first but building over time to not being able to concentrate on complicated written material or wanting to take a rest, a power nap, during the afternoon.

They find food allergies where they previously did not have them.

Hormonal issues for ladies may have become more pronounced.

Allergic reactions like hay fever or sensitivity to animal hair/fur are worse than they were or may arise even though you have not had that problem before

There can be sensitivity to colds and Flu and when someone near you has something rather than you just net getting it you find that you seem to be catching everyone else's conditions.

Lack of motivation to do things that you previously did, especially sport and events that require social interaction – basically the feeling that you just could not be bothered and that you just want to rest or sleep.

Often they do not think there is anything specifically wrong but they know that things are not 'right'.

At this stage of CFS there needs to be care taken before putting labels on things. It may be that you have just been working really hard, or that there is stress in your life from your work or from family situations and that you just need a good rest.

Telling the difference from just being run down and to having onset CFS is a challenge in the early stages.

One lady I spoke with said that she used to go and do the shopping and bring it all home and put it all away and then have a cup of tea. Nowadays she was finding that she would do the shopping and bring it home and have to sit and have a cup of tea _before_ she had the energy to put the shopping away.

There was nothing specific that was wrong but she knew that things were not the way they were, things were not 'right' and she could not find anyone to adviser on what should could do about it.

Someone once explained to me that they felt it was like a dream where there is a black cloud behind them that is getting closer and closer and no matter what they did they could feel it approaching.

'Black cloud' was the term they used as there was nothing specific that they could find that they could deal with and it created a feeling of discomfort and powerlessness.

Interestingly this is very similar to the sort of feeling of impending doom that is closely related to people with depression.

If you are a person who is showing signs of slipping into CFS then I suggest you get hold of nutrition products like described here and use them as a nutritional supplement.

It is wise to begin with an Amino-protein shake and a set of tablets just once a day for a couple of days.

While you are using this you can be adding Aloe Vera juice to your water and sipping it through the day. Water use in the first few weeks is very important as you will be detoxifying chemicals from your body and the water helps to flush those poisons out of you.

If you are using the aloe then you will be healing and cleansing through your bowel at the same time. I recommend that at the very least you get a 1 litre/2 pint drink bottle, fill with clean water and aloe juice, and sip it constantly throughout the day.

These things will begin the detoxification process to let the body start to cleanse itself and also allow the system to adjust to the nutrition that is being added into the diet.

After a day or two, if there are no problems, then the shake can be added to your daily program, to be taken a couple of times a day and the tablets can be taken 3 times a day, which is the normal recommended use of the products.

This enables your body to get its nutrition and cleansing in 5 hour blocks.

Using the products I recommended the Amino-Protein Shake (I will just call it Shake from here on) is soy based and will not affect lactose intolerance. Protein being soy based generally does not have issues for Celiac conditions either.

If you can eat normal food and eat a sandwich with bread and filling then the nutrition products are just food and you should have no problem with them.

In this case you can decide what products you want to use. The 4 I listed previously are best: Shake, multivitamin, Aloe Vera and acidophilus fiber tablets.

I believe that this 90 day cycle is critical to establish a firm foundation for your health. You may get good results in a week but it has taken a long time for your CFS to develop and you should not be expecting it to clear up overnight.

In around 90 days your whole blood volume will basically be replaced with new cells. That is a great time frame to feed your body good nutrition and get yourself back on a good health footing.

The shake and multivitamin products will assist with villi rebuild by themselves. Adding the aloe and acidophilus fiber tablets is better. Anything more that than that is up to you but is not required, in my opinion, for dealing directly with your CFS.

Superfoods that Fight Chronic Fatigue
Syndrome

If you are seriously working on dealing with your CFS then concentrate on that initially. If you are also interested in using dietary supplements for weight control then that's great but for now let's get you well and you can then look at using supplements for changing weight and resizing once you have your health in order.

How To Use The Products - Level 1 CFS

The best way is to just start on the program you choose and to then use it in the way the instructions recommend.

That should be that you take at least one shake a day and the tablet supplements 3 times a day (when you would normally eat).

It is great to start the day with a shake. You can add it to your breakfast or replace your breakfast with just the shake and tabs.

2 shakes are better than one so if you add a second shake into your diet at lunch of in the evening that that is better. It is not critical, the process of rebuilding villi should happen with one shake but taking 2 should give you quicker results.

The second shake should be added with your lunch or after work before or after dinner.

It is your choice whether or not you choose to have more than 1 shake a day.

Think of the tablets as herbs and leaves, twigs and berries all chopped up really fine and mixed in the right proportions then pressed into tablet form to make it easy to take them.

Herbs get into your system fast and the out of your system fast so you are looking at taking them regularly throughout your day. The best guide is to take them at normal meal times.

Quantity for the shake powder is 2 scoops per serve. If you do not have a scoop supplied then one scoop is equivalent to 2 flat desert spoons (1 rounded desert spoon).

The shake needs to be one that you really like. You need to like the flavor and look forward to taking it.

For that reason, when you are offered a choice of flavors for the shake I recommend that people use a Berry flavor as it can be quite simple, even mixed with water, and taste good.

Don't make the mistake of thinking that shake means Milk shake. It is important that you are not taking the shake in milk or skim milk initially.

Let me repeat that last statement to be very clear: at least until you are experiencing really good health results, and your condition has improved and stabilized, I would like you not to use cow's milk as the foundation for your shake.

That is not to say you need to cut milk out of your diet. What you take now: milk in coffee or tea, on cereal etc is fine. Just don't _add_ a large hit of milk into your diet with the shake.

Soy Milk should be fine and rice milk is okay if that is what you like.

I prefer that you mix the shake in water. I use about 300-400 ml of water in mine.

It is much nicer to drink very cold, with iced water or with ice added.

You might like to use some fruit juice with it but bear in mind that commercial fruit juice is packed full of sugar. If you wanted the sweetness in the shake then a little juice, water and ice would work.

We want it to taste great so you feel good about using it but we want it to be healthy.

If you have time then mixing it in a blender is a great idea as you can add some fresh fruit to it and blend in some ice. Putting frozen berries in water with ice and your shake powder makes a really nice shake.

If you are working to find something that suits you then you can even mix the shake powder into yoghurt. Using commercial flavored yoghurt means you are adding sugars and chemicals but overall that is not likely to be a problem and getting your shake to something you really like is more important initially.

If you are blending you can even drop a little yoghurt into the blender to make it more creamy.

At this point we have things moving forward: when you have your nutrition products in hand and you have a few ways to mix your shake that you really like then your job is really done.

The task then is to stay on the products and let your body heal itself.

Elite athletes, who also pay a lot of attention to what they eat, normally feel and energy shift within a few hours of using products like this.

For normal healthy people we expect to see a measurable shift in personal energy levels in about 3 days.

For people with mild CFS I am looking for results but are really expecting to see at least 1 good day in 7 to 10 days from starting.

I am not looking for instant wellness and I have said often in the book that we are not trying to 'cure'. We are giving the body the tools to heal itself.

Superfoods that Fight Chronic Fatigue Syndrome

When you get 1 good day, then you know you are on the right track and that your health is on an upward path at last.

Remember that I have said that you should commit yourself to 90 days on products.

If you feel great after 3 days do not think you are better.

It took an extended time for your CFS to develop and to think it has cleared up after a very short time, even if you Do Feel a lot better is asking too much. Be gentle and patient with yourself.

If you are not experiencing at least 1 good day within the first 10 days I would be asking you why you are mixing your shake in milk (as that would be the most common factor that would impede your recovery).

Of course the other factor is not actually taking the products as they do not work if you leave them in the containers. I will assume though that if you have taken the time to research this, read this book, found the products and actually have them in your hands and that you will go on and use them as directed.

At the end of this section I will go through what to expect as you use the products so you can be watching for things that may happen and recognize them, embrace them as positive signs of improving health, and know how to work with them.

First though I want to go through how to use the products for people with more serious health issues.

Level 2. Established Chronic Fatigue Syndrome

As the condition worsens your body tries to reduce energy expenditure and so things related to low metabolic rate appear.

This group will often find:

Lack of concentration where things you read or try to understand just do not 'stick' in your mind. You review material or read something and 10 minutes later you just cannot remember what it is about.

Weariness that may find them falling asleep whenever they stop actively doing things.

Short periods of the day when there is energy to do things and blocks of the day when motivation and energy are extremely low. Often people in this group will start setting aside things like cooking a meal and they just cannot organize and motivate themselves to do it.

Advanced food allergies that often require careful attention to diet.

Lack of energy that makes it extremely hard to get out of bed in the mornings.

Superfoods that Fight Chronic Fatigue Syndrome

Often people in this group with have sort medical advice and initially been directed to supplements and tonics because there is no specific illness that is able to be identified. As the condition develops further medical advice may have established that a CFS condition is present and rest, low stress environment, good nutrition and maybe vitamin and mineral supplements have been recommended.

For people who have been dealing with the problem of CFS for some time and are showing the signs that are recognized as being associated with it, but who are still able to function with a basically normal life, then we should still be a little cautious when starting on nutrition supplements.

I am now talking about people who have had the condition for over a long period and the longer term effects of lowered immune system and lowered metabolic rate are becoming apparent.

In these case there is likely to be food intolerances. Using quality nutrition products should not cause any harm but with a low immune system and fragile metabolisms then "change of diet" is always something to approach carefully.

There is likely to also be the obvious problem with fatigue that we have come to associate with CFS. We expect this to turn around with the right nutrition program.

It is something that will have ups and downs and there will still be good days and bad days but within a period of a few weeks we are expecting that the good days are more common.

Within 6 weeks or so I normally find that the bad days are now better than the good days used to be. Improvement seems to be a bit erratic as you live thought it but the process of improvement is an upward slope that keeps getting better.

If there is any sign of the body reacting to the nutrition products then look through the section on "What to expect when you get started."

Level 2 - How to take supplements

If you are in this group then I would expect that you have already had to make changes in the way you live so that you can still function, and undertake the tasks of normal daily life, while working around the CFS.

People with this CFS this far advanced normally would be expected to have food allergies and diet difficulties.

Specific food intolerances like Celiac Disease are not generally directly linked with CFS but as your whole immune system slows and begins to falter then dietary issues become more common. If you have some allergy tests I expect you will find a whole range of foods that show negative reactions.

As you slip further with your CFS then more and more foods you will be show up as foods you are allergic to or at least intolerant of. That leads to people adjusting their diets and restricting what they eat.

This is just a reality of living with CFS. If you fit into this category then I expect that for you it is already part of your own personal reality.

As we work with nutritional supplements I suggest that you treat these allergies and intolerances as _symptoms_ of your CFS and not as actual problems in their own right.

When we get your system working again then you will find that most of the problems you are trying to deal with on a day by day basis will improve

(Again I ask you to create a list of all the things that are currently wrong with your health and appearance before you begin using nutrition products so you can remember what it was like before you started.

This will be important to you as you progressively improve. On that list make sure you add all the foods that you cannot now comfortably eat. As you improve I expect that one by one you will find these foods are no longer problems for you.)

One of the main questions that people with more advanced CFS normally have in the front of their mind is if there is anything in the nutrition products that will give bad reactions with their food allergies.

The answer to that is that used properly you should be able to avoid having issues.

Even people with Celiac and lactose issues should have no problem using products if they pay attention and follow some simple steps.

Nutrition products like the ones I recommend are food products, not medications, and are not contraindicated with general medications. That means if you can eat an apple without that effecting any medication you are on you should be able to use nutrition products.

If you have doubts though you should then either take the product itself, or a copy of the label showing ingredients, to your doctor, or other health professional you are working with, and ask if there are any problems using them.

Your question for them needs to be: "Is there anything in this product that would be harmful for me?"

In most cases you will find that the medical professional is not in a position to endorse use of nutritional products but they should be able to look at the labels of any product and be able to tell you that they will not do you any harm.

Medical professionals with a strong interest in their patients and their profession often ask if they can monitor your progress on the products to ensure you keep as well as you can.

Level 3 & 4. Severe Chronic Fatigue Syndrome Symptoms

When the CFS really sets in people find their life just falls to pieces.

I knew a lady, Karen, who had diagnosed with CFS and had a team of specialists watching over her. She was really bad and I will tell her story as it gives an idea of just where you can get to if the CFS is allowed to run its path.

She found that she was not living in the city as she was too sensitive to environmental toxins. I am not just talking about air pollution. She was not able to handle being in a room with products made from petro-carbons which, of course, includes plastics.

She could not stay in a room where there was a lot of plastics. If she entered a room where there had been aerosol sprays used in the last few days she had an immediate reaction.

132

Her food intolerances were massive and specialist dieticians were working with her to identify her allergies and foods she could not eat. The end result of that was that she was living on a range of 5 different vegetables and filtered water and that was all that she could handle.

Her food intolerance was so bad that if she ate anything with yeast in it then within 10 minutes she would have a reaction that was so bad that all colour would drain from her face and she would go dead white.

Her face and her throat would swell up so badly that she would have to be laid down with her shoulders elevated and her head back to open her airways enough to allow her to continue breathing.

That is an extreme case of CFS but it is not an isolated case.

I mention this case mainly for people who are dealing with a more mild condition so they are aware of just how bad things can become over time with CFS left untreated.

In the same note I will give further feedback on Karen so you can see there is light at the end of the tunnel.

She used the nutrition products we talk about here and over a period of 8 or 9 months pulled back from the health problems so that she could get back to living a normal life.

I had a fair amount of contact with her as she was a resource in that she was always happy to help advise and support other people who had CFS problems to help guide them back to health.

I lost contact with Karen for some time then bumped into her in the city. It was lunch time and grabbed lunch together. She ate pizza without any problem as gave thanks again for her recovery.

She was working as a personal assistant for the head of a brewery where the air was full of yeast. She said that when she was at her worst just walking past that building would have put here in hospital but now she worked there every day without a problem.

When people have more advanced severe chronic fatigue syndrome symptoms then there are normally food allergies like lactose (milk) intolerance and Celiac Disease (Wheat and gluten intolerance), and similar conditions.

The food allergies are part and parcel of the condition and they do should not present a major problem with a nutrition program like this but you need to pay attention and show some common sense.

If there is any chance that the condition has roots in chemical contamination, or drug use, or if it is just a fully developed case of chronic fatigue syndrome then the sufferer already knows that they have serious problems and that it not going to sort itself out overnight.

In extreme cases it is best to use just one of products for the first few days, or even a week, to ensure that your body is comfortable with it and to begin a gentle detoxification process.

In severe cases of CFS then the first product to use is simply Aloe Vera Juice diluted in water.

How To Use Nutritional Supplement Products if you think you have a more advanced, Level 3 or 4 CFS condition.

In your case, as your system is more sensitive to change I recommend you be a lot more methodical and more patient in your approach to using the nutrition products, and I recommend that you introduce them over a period of time.

As I have said, your condition took a long time to become established, applying patience in turning it around to ensure you get a solid and permanent result just makes sense.

While a normal healthy person would use one or two shakes a day along with vitamin and mineral supplementation from the very start, I do not recommend that for you, as you have the allergy and food sensitivity issues that they do not.

In your case I recommend that it is best to begin by using the Aloe Vera juice and the Acidophilus products that you begin with them just once a day for a couple of days.

What we are doing here is generating a mild cleansing program.

The use of Aloe Vera and Acidophilus fiber tablets is designed to generate a gentle detoxification process to clean your bowel and to begin your body gently removing toxins and poisons from your system, without overloading your ability to clear those toxins out from your bloodstream.

As we have discussed earlier, many people with advanced CFS are finically challenged as they have not been able to do full time work.

(It is best, in my opinion, to use the Aloe Vera and Acidophilus fiber tablets but it is not critical. If you situation precludes you from using these products then skip this next section and go straight to the section below on using the Amino-protein shake and vitamin and mineral tablets but if you are going to do that them please take additional time to slowly introduce products to ensure that we have every chance of turning your health around. Be patient and take small steps.)

Directions for how much Aloe Vera to use are on the container. Initially it is good if you take one serve over a day. If you are using the concentrate you may like to add it to your water bottle and drink it over the day.

The same applies for non-concentrated aloe or even aloe in the powder from if that is available in your country. If it is not convenient to add it into drink over the day then you can use maybe a third of a serve each of 3 times during the day.

You can mix the aloe in water or with another liquid. If you use juices in your normal diet then just add it to the juice if you like. Any cold drink is fine to add the aloe to. I always look for ways that people enjoy using their nutrition products so they look forward to taking them.

Often people say "I am used to doing what I have to do with my health and if it will help then it does not matter what something tastes like".

The reality is that if you like the taste of something and you can feel it doing good for you then you will take into your lifestyle as part of your diet and that is the outcome we want – Take the time and the effort to find a way that you really enjoy using the products you take.

With this low level introduction of Aloe Vera I would not expect much reaction. This is for people who have really sensitive systems and working slowly through using products is worthwhile if the end result is that you are feeling well all the time.

Be patient with the process. We are not looking for instant results here but for sustainable, permanent, improvement and it is worth taking it in gentle steps.

If in the first day you do not have a reaction to the Aloe Vera then on day two take it up to normal use and have the Aloe Vera juice 2 or 3 times during the day, again, mixed in whatever you like.

If there are no problems with that then it is time to move on.

If there you have any reaction to the aloe then the worst I would expect is a little bit of diarrhea or an unsettled stomach and that should settle in a day or so.

With any nutrition product like this it is best for people with allergies and more serious health issues to introduce them one at a time and start on minimum use and then build up. If you have any adverse reaction, then pull back from using that product and work with the others you have.

You can try reintroducing the initial product in a week or two. It often seems amazing that once we get your health improving just how quickly your body will strengthen and allow you to go back to eating things you previously had difficulty with.

Once you are comfortable with the Aloe Vera then you should begin the Acidophilus fiber tablets.

Normal use for that would be one tablet 3 times a day. Generally that is taken at normal meal times.

Initially I would like you to use just one tablet, once. Not take any more in the first day.

Again, like the Aloe Vera, I do not expect any reaction to this tablet but CFS can be very sensitive and we want to be very methodical in introducing anything into your system.

Adding one product at a time means you can clear monitor everything you are doing and if there is anything among the products that you do have a reaction to then you will know exactly what it is an be able to work with it.

You will not need to stop everything as you probably would if you were not doing this gentle introduction of one product at a time.

As the Acidophilus fiber tablets will absorb liquids it is best to separate using liquid Aloe Vera from taking the Acidophilus fiber tablet so that it does not absorb the Aloe Vera and pass it out of your system. Something like 20 min separation should be fine.

As the Acidophilus fiber tablet will absorb water you would normally take it with a large glass of water.

If you had any problem with diarrhea or lose bowel movements then take it with little water and it will assist with absorbing fluid from the bowel.

If you are constipated then use more water and the fiber in the tablet will help to loosen bowel motions.

If you do not find any issues in the first day then take the Acidophilus fiber tablet morning and night the next day and then go on to tablets 3 times a day.

Now we will deal with the core products in the nutrition program being recommended.

They are the Amino-protein shake and multivitamin supplements.

More Tips For Using an Amino-protein Shake in Your CFS Diet.

The way to use the shake is to begin by taking a very small serve, once in a day.

I said earlier that normal use is about 4 flat desert spoons. Initially I recommend that you take just one teaspoon of shake only. Put that into a liquid that you are familiar and comfortable with.

This gives you a chance to ensure that you have no problems with the shake.

In such small quantities we would expect no reaction but we do this so we can be sure that it is okay.

If that is fine then the next day try taking the teaspoon of shake powder a couple of times in the say or increase the use to a dessertspoon of shake powder.

If at any time you are uncomfortable with using the products then stop. Wait a couple of days and then try again at this very low level.

If you are also using the Aloe and Acidophilus fiber tablets then you will find that a few days more will assist in building your system and when you reintroduce the shake powder it is likely that you will find it is no longer a problem.

You will be familiar with the introduction of a new product I expect so you can do this at your own speed. What I am looking for is a very gentle introduction so that you are comfortable with the products and so you do not get an initial bad reaction.

Superfoods that Fight Chronic Fatigue Syndrome

We also do not want to trigger detoxification to a level where you have that additional pressure on your system.

Some people will bring their shake use up to normal levels in just a couple of days.

Others could take a week.

There is no race to get things going. The more difficulty you have with your health the more important it is that we find a long term solution for you.

It has taken a long time to fall from good health to where you are now and you can expect to spend some time to get back to what can be considered as normal health.

As you build your use of the Amino-protein shake powder you may like to move to half strength shakes twice a day.

For our purposes in trying to trigger rebuilding of your ingestion that half strength shake, 2 flat dessertspoon/1 scoop, will be quite effective.

When you are comfortable with taking the Amino-protein shake powder then it is time to add the multivitamins to bring yourself up to a full basic program.

We do this the same way: take one tablet, once, and wait till the next day.

Adding one product at a time allows you to see how each one works for you and if there is any discomfort you know exactly what your body is reacting to.

If you find any discomfort with the multivitamin tablets then stop using them and just take the other products for a couple of days then try them again.

When you are comfortable we are looking to build this product use to one tablet, three times a day.

When you have introduced all these products then you are doing your job, we now need to wait on your body taking this nutrition and using it to cleanse and to rebuild.

In that process you will detoxify chemicals so keeping your water use up to a high level in these first few weeks is a priority.

Best medical advice is that you should be drinking daily:

1 quart of water for every 55 lb of body weight. (1 lt of water for every 25kg of body weight)

For most of us this seems like a lot and I am not going to tell you to drink this amount of water for the rest of your life, just make sure you have higher than normal water use for the first few weeks of using products.

Some of the more obvious signs of your body detoxifying chemicals out of your body include:

Dull headache like a hangover
Muscle stiffness, especially in shoulders and back (feeling a bit like you have muscle fatigue after weight training)
Dizziness
Bad breath and/or body odour
Skin breakout (pimples etc)

How long is it going to take before I feel better, when using natural nutritional supplements?

For some people using the product brand that I recommend, they will get a result in just a couple of days! Elite spots people often feel a difference in their bodies within a few hours.

Normal healthy people would expect to feel an energy shift in about 3 days as their body rebuilds its ability to absorb nutrition and use the nutrition you are giving it.

For people in this group I hope to see a response within 7 to 10 days. If we do get a measurable energy shift within the first 10 days then you can be fairly sure that the path to recovery will be fairly constant, with good days and bad days but a steady upwards trend back to having control of your health.

If you have not found changes in the first 10 days then the next group of people tend to see that breakthrough at around 6 or 7 weeks. Quite often these people are people who have had some viral infection or other serious health challenges associated with their CFS.

While these is a clear pattern in that case it is less than 10% of the people who I have dealt with who have CFS that take this long to get measurable positive responses to product use.

The final group would be maybe 5% who have had chemical contamination.

Advanced CFS Sufferers May Take Longer To Feel The Difference

If you fall into this group then we have to expect that you have had a virus problem that has affected your immune system or you have an underlying chemical contamination problem with chemicals still in your system.

Go back to the Level 2 - Established CFS section above and go through the steps of how to use the products listed there.

Superfoods that Fight Chronic Fatigue Syndrome

For people with established CFS these are suggestions to work with. If you fall into this final 5% or 10% of CFS sufferers then the guidelines of how to slowly introduce the products are not optional, they are critical.

You have already tried everything you have been able to find to turn your CFS around and most of what we have said here will align with what you have found in the past. You would not introduce anything into your diet without caution and care.

The slow introduction listed above may take you a week or two to establish full product use. No problem.

You have been a long time getting to where you are now and it will not turn around overnight, you know that. Just be careful in getting started on the nutrition products.

For people at your level you are not expecting miracles, in fact it is likely that you do not believe you will ever find an answer. I have no problems with that either.

What I do point out is that you cannot say that you have tried everything till you have tried this as well and, obviously; I believe you have found your answers here and, God willing, you will see recovery.

Just take your time introducing products and stay with it.

For people who have had a bad viral infection it can be 6 weeks till you get that first 'good day'. People with chemical issues can take up to the full 90 days to have that first really 'good day' and it may not be an easy journey.

Chemical contaminated people will know that things are happening though. People with CFS at this level are normally very aware of everything they do and how things affect their body and their condition. They have to be aware in self-defense as if they get things wrong they can spend days, even weeks, in bed recovering from their mistake.

These people will know that things are happening when they get on nutrition products as there will be change. The one outcome I do not want to see is NO change. If your body is beginning to deal with the issues then things will happen for the better.

I have seen several cases where people have been sure they are regressing and the whole project is going badly as the health issues that they have dealt with previously and gotten under control can manifest again.

One of the first people I worked with was very unhappy with this reoccurring of past health issues but she was strong in her will to find an answer and knew that something was happening and so she stuck with the products.

After a couple of weeks she realized, to her amazement, that the problems she was experiencing was like a mirror image of problems she had dealt with in the past, working backwards through the history of what she had been through. Like she was peeling the layers of an onion, dealing with previous health issues one-by-one, back in time.

When she had worked through those issues, about 8 weeks, she finally had one day when she woke up in the morning feeling rested and alive for the first day in many years. She was first up in the house and did jobs and made breakfast.

He husband thought there must have been burglars and came out to face them as he could not conceive that she had got up before him as that had not happened in many years.

What I am saying is that CFS can be a perplexing condition and we are not looking to cure anything, we are giving your body the tools it can use to cure itself. There is no clear path of recovery where you can just tick the boxes one after the other.

You will need to do your part in giving your body the tools it needs to heal and allow it to do so in its own time.

Next I will share with you some of the more popular recipes that people have shared when they explored the many ways to create delicious meals from their shake powder.

Finding the most tasty and enjoyable ways to take your nutrition is key to your success in a CFS diet therapy.

If you don't like the taste or enjoy your daily food you won't stick to the nutritional therapy, so keep trying all combinations to make sure you have a delicious variety of flavours in your shakes to enjoy every day.

Popular Shake Recipes

You can mix your Amino-Protein Powder into a shake in any way you like. If you want to get adventurous then there are basically no limits to tasty and enjoyable ways to take it.

Here are a range of suggestions that you would probably never think of if you did not have something to begin to trigger your thinking:

"BERRY CHEESECAKE" Shake

1/2 Small tub Chobani Greek yoghurt - Strawberry flavour, fat-free
2 scoops Vanilla Amino-Protein Powder
1 scoop Berry Amino-Protein Powder

Superfoods that Fight Chronic Fatigue
Syndrome

350ml coconut water
1 tablespoon organic Coconut Oil
2 soup spoons frozen organic berries
2-3 ice cubes
Blend thoroughly.

Lemon Snack

1 x Greek Yoghurt (Non-Fat Plain flavour, 150g tub)
3 x Scoops Vanilla Amino-Protein Powder
Juice of half a Lemon
Cut off some Lemon Rind (few pieces of 'zest')
2 ice cubes
Blend up in your rocket-blender! Oh my Goodness!
Tastes like Lemon Cheesecake!

To make Shake Version:

1 x Greek Yoghurt tub (as per above)
3 x Scoops Vanilla Amino-Protein Powder
Juice of half a Lemon
Add some Lemon Zest (1/2 of the used 1/2 of lemon
- add to blender)
300ml Water

Yummy Berry Mousse

200ml water (or soy milk)
3 ice cubes
3 scoops Berry Amino-Protein Powder
Handful of frozen berries

Blend and eat!!

Strawberry & Cream

3 Scoops of Berry Amino-Protein Powder
300 mls Water (or low fat milk / low fat soy milk)
5-10 Strawberries
2 Tablespoons Non-Fat GREEK YogHurt
Blend & enjoy!!

Protein Pancakes

1/3 cup of wholemeal self raising flour (or gluten free if you prefer)
1 egg,
3/4 cup of soy milk,
1 Scoop of Vanilla Amino-Protein Powder and
1 Chocolate Amino-Protein Powder

Yummmmmm

Practical tips for planning how to get your new nutrition into your daily routines.

By regularly changing your rice/soy milk flavours eg: strawberry, chocolate, vanilla, berry, fruits, caramel, coffee, you can get whatever milk shake flavours you like that way, and change the flavours every few days to keep the shakes interesting to drink.

The booklet enclosed with your protein shake products will give you some recipe & fruit mix 'thick shake' ideas to try out. If you find the shakes are too thick for you to enjoy, add more water, or use slightly less powder.

You should have at least one heaped dessertspoon of powder in one 250ml / cup of Shake drink.

For simple daily shakes you can pre-mix your shake powder, water, and soy milk in the evening before you go to bed.

Just shake and put in the fridge overnight. That way the powder dissolves overnight and with a couple of quick shakes it makes a smooth drink without taking any time for blenders etc. in the morning rush hour.

And if you go out to work every day, you just mix a double serve the night before and take the rest of the pre-mixed shake to work in a bottle or cool thermos and drink it at lunchtime.

For a leisurely lunch fruit smoothie I will take one of the recipes and mix the fresh fruit and other ingredients in a blender. Very nice when I make the time to do this.

To drink 2 quarts/liters of water with aloe juice added (throughout the day) you keep a 1 quart/ltr squeezie plastic pop-top bottle that you can drink from throughout the day, as well as when you take your tablets.

You can buy some screw on pop tops and put them on the actual bottle the Aloe juice comes in as it has a great consistency to 'squeeze' my water aloe juice mix out from as I drive and rush around.

In the beginning you may like to save a half serve of shake (1/2 cup - 125ml) to take before you go to bed at night, as a Supper snack.

This gives your body good nutrition to work on and absorb when you sleep, so that when you wake up in the morning you already well fed and energized.

Bear in mind the principle that for optimum nutritional benefit your body needs a small serve of nutrition every 5 hours.

If you want to lose some weight and trim your fat intake levels while you are working on improving your overall health then you can replace two meals with the shakes.

Now that you have the knowledge of how to cleanse your body of toxins and help it rebuild your villi to be better able to absorb the nutrition from the food you eat, you can start to discover what the most powerful superfoods are that will help you to eat yourself healthy again.

In the next chapter we will look at the top superfoods and learn about each of their particular properties that you can target to improve your own healthy to beat CFS.

Many of these fruits, berries and vegetables are perfect to be incorporated into your daily shake nutrition drink.

Now that you have addressed your body's ability to absorb the nutrition you feed it, you can look at the best power packed foods that you can select to design yourself a CFS diet, which is what we will cover in the next chapter.

Chapter Six:
Superfoods that Fight Chronic Fatigue Syndrome – and Provide Overall Wellness

Once your body is finally able to once again fully absorb the good nutrition you provide it, it's important to make sure you incorporate the most powerful foods on earth that are going to go to work for you in the fight against Chronic Fatigue Syndrome.

There are many foods that have properties and nutrients that help restore a healthy immune system, energy, and have anti-inflammatory properties. In this section you'll learn about some specific foods you need to add to your CFS diet.

Almost any fruit or vegetable is going to have special nutrients that make it healthy for you. But here we'll highlight some of the most important ones and discuss some other types of foods that can be considered superfoods.

Superfoods that Fight Chronic Fatigue Syndrome

The idea of superfoods originally came from Dr. Nicholas Perricone's list of 10 top superfoods.

Since that time the list has been expanded to include many foods that contain antioxidants and other important nutrients and help to calm inflammation.

Let's look at some of the top superfoods to immediately add to your daily CFS diet!

Fruits and Berries

There are many fruits and berries that can have an incredible impact on your health and wellness.

Make sure to include them when you're writing out your grocery list. Fruits and berries are tasty treats that also pack a powerful nutritional punch.

When possible, buy organic produce or grow your own to ensure it's free from toxins. It's also best to buy foods in season so that you get high quality nutrition from them. It's also important to eat a large variety.

The more colorful your diet is, the more of the nutrients you're getting. So balancing out your plate to have greens, reds, yellows, oranges, and blues means you'll have more balanced nutrition.

Red Grapes

Red grapes are full of antioxidants that can help you to fight inflammation and the effect of toxins in the environment.

This includes eating actual grapes, drinking grape juice, and even the effects of red wine. In fact, grape juice will provide you with more concentrated nutrients than the grapes alone.

Research conducted in France has shown that red wine actually can add years to your life if you limit your use to one or two glasses per day. Drinking more than that can actually take years off of your life.

The nutrients found in red grapes include manganese, potassium, vitamin C, and manganese.

In addition to fighting CFS, red grapes can help you to prevent cancer, heart disease, and Alzheimer's disease.

Blueberries

Blueberries also contain high levels of antioxidants. Research from Tufts University found that eating a half cup of blueberries daily can actually prevent problems with dementia and memory.

These antioxidants help to fight inflammation and repair damage done by stress that can be related to CFS.

When choosing berries, make sure to look for the darkest ones so that you get the most anti-oxidants.

Oranges

Many people depend on vitamin C supplements to help keep their immune system strong. But you'll actually get more benefit from eating oranges or drinking a glass of orange juice each day.

Oranges contain a lot of vitamin C, and in the fruit or juice your body is also given important properties to absorb the vitamin better. Oranges are important for building a healthy immune system.

It also helps to build strong ligaments helping your joints to be healthier. In addition to helping your fight against CFS, they can also help you to have a healthier heart and lower risk of developing cancer.

Apples

The saying "an apple a day keeps the doctor away" could be true! These little gems are easy to grab on the go and are also full of antioxidants such as vitamin C, potassium, and flavonoids. They're also full of fiber which means healthy digestion.

Make sure that you eat the skin – that's where most of the antioxidants are stored.

Also make sure and eat a variety of different apples because they have a variety of different nutrients to share with you.

Avocado

Avocados are full of healthy fat that keeps your heart happy. Healthy fat is also good for the nervous system and helps to maintain healthy connections between your neurons. This is very beneficial for someone suffering from CFS.

Beyond the nutrients that it contains, avocados have been shown to actually help you absorb the nutrients from your food better.

So it's a great addition to a salad or other nutrient-rich meal to help your body get the best of what you're giving to it.

Tufts University researchers also found that eating avocado can help to improve the health of your brain.

In addition, avocado can help to prevent cancer and heart disease when made a regular part of a healthy diet.

Superfoods that Fight Chronic Fatigue Syndrome

Pomegranate

When summer ends it can be a sad time for fruit enthusiasts. But the pomegranate helps to bring a little extra joy to the autumn season. This is a fruit that's chock full of vitamins and minerals.

It's full of antioxidants that can help to prevent heart disease and reduce inflammation in the body.

You can drink the juice of the pomegranate to get some of the nutrients or you can eat the seeds themselves.

When you open a large, heavy pomegranate you'll reveal hundreds of little tasty seeds.

It's a little bit of work to expose the edible part of the fruit, but it's well worth it for the nutritional benefits as well as the taste.

Tomatoes

Tomatoes contain the nutrient lycopene that's a super nutrient. A diet high in lycopene can help to reduce your risk of cancer by as much as 40%.

You'll also help to prevent heart disease and improve the health of your nervous system.

Not only can you enjoy benefits from eating tomatoes themselves, you'll also get benefits from eating tomato products such as tomato sauce and salsa.

In fact, sauces will provide you with a concentrated amount of lycopene.

CamuCamu berries

You may never have heard of these berries, but camucamu berries are berries that provide many antioxidants and can help to fight inflammation in the body. They're very high in vitamin C and can strengthen the immune system.

They also can help to keep your blood sugar stabilized. Most people don't eat the berries whole because they're quite sour in taste. However, you can get camu juice and it can be found in powder and capsule form.

Acai Berries

Acai berries hail from South America where they've been eaten for centuries. But now acai berries are marketed as a superfood – and for good reason.

They're full of antioxidants that help to prevent disease and calm inflammation in the body.

They're high in vitamins, minerals, fiber, plant sterols, and contain healthy fats. While they were once difficult to find, they're becoming much more common and can be found in many supermarkets and health food stores.

Superfoods that Fight Chronic Fatigue Syndrome

You may also be able to find acai berry supplements and juices. However, it's best to eat the actual berry to get all of the nutrition from it.

Figs

Figs have been eaten since ancient times in the Middle East. They grow from fig trees and are small with a thin skin and fruit with tiny seeds inside.

They're sometimes overlooked when thinking about superfoods, but they definitely fit that status.

Figs are high in calcium, fiber, and plant nutrients that help to prevent cancer, diabetes, chronic diseases, and infections. They also contain chlorogenic acid.

This is an important substance that helps to control blood sugar. It can enhance your weight loss efforts and help you to have more energy.

Gojiberries

Goji berries are native to China and the Himalayas. They have antioxidants that help to protect you from disease and slow down the aging process.

They also contain lyceum barbarum polysaccharides. This is the scientific name for a type of sugar that helps you to improve immunity by helping cells to communicate better with each other.

You can find goji berries in many health food stores. You may also be able to find goji juice, though it's better to eat the berries. They can be eaten the same way you eat other berries or raisins.

Lemon

Lemons are fairly common fruits that frequently are overlooked because of how common they are. However, there are many reasons to squeeze a little extra juice into your water or add it to a recipe.

Just as oranges improve immunity, so do other citrus fruits, such as lemons. In addition, lemons can help to lower your blood pressure and prevent cancer.

They also contain antioxidants to protect you from disease and slow down the effects of aging and toxins.

You'll also appreciate that lemon juice can be used to treat inflammation making it a powerful weapon against autoimmune diseases and chronic disease. It also helps to prevent dehydration and can help to improve digestion.

Lemon juice can be added to beverages or recipes in order for you to get the benefits.

Juice can also be used as a mouthwash to freshen your breath and kill bacteria in your mouth or applied to skin to treat acne and dry skin.

Superfoods that Fight Chronic Fatigue Syndrome

Mangos

Mango is a fruit native to South America that has been enjoyed there for ages. But many people outside of that region are beginning to discover the delicious taste and health benefits of a juicy mango.

Mangos help to improve your digestion because of their fiber content and also a particular enzyme they contain that helps to promote healthy digestion.

They contain vitamins and minerals that improve your heart health and prevent disease as well.

In addition, mangoes are high in vitamin A, making them a good food for improving your eye health and vision.

And if you're having problems with hormones and sex drive, eating mangos may be the perfect antidote.

Mangos are delicious fruits that contain a yellow fruit beneath the peal. The fruit may be eaten as is or added to sauces, salsas, and meats.

Cantaloupe

You may not know it, but cantaloupe is one of the fruits highest in vitamin C. By eating one cup of it you'll get all you need for the day of vitamins A and C.

It helps to improve the quality of your skin and helps to improve your immune system to fight infection.

They help to prevent cancer, heart disease, and support good eye health.

They're full of water which helps to prevent problems with dehydration in a hot climate. These melons are also easy to find, inexpensive, and easy to eat.

Cherries

Cherries are delicious fruits that have many health benefits. Like many fruits and berries, they contain antioxidants to help slow aging and protect you from toxins and the effects of the sun.

They also work to reduce inflammation which can help improve problems such as arthritis, diabetes, and heart disease.

In fact, they're pain relievers much like an anti-inflammatory medication you might buy.

Another interesting health benefit of cherries is that they help you to get a good night's sleep.

They contain the natural hormone called melatonin that your body uses to promote sleep.

Eating cherries regularly can help you with sleep problems that are common to Chronic Fatigue

Syndrome. You'll find that your sleep becomes more routine and you're able to rest better.

Coconut

Coconuts a grown from trees in tropical regions. They are known for having many healthful properties in the coconut flesh, the coconut water, coconut cream, and coconut oil they contain.

Coconuts are high in fiber as well as other vitamins and minerals. They also contain healthy fats and electrolytes.

You can now purchase coconut water marketed specifically to help replenish your body's potassium and sodium.

The meat of the coconut is just under the hard shell. It is high in manganese which helps you to have a better metabolism and it can help to support healthy blood sugar levels in the body.

This lowers your risk of diabetes and heart disease. Coconut can also be helpful in weight loss efforts.

It's important when you eat coconut, that you eat it in the purest form rather than coconut that has added sugar.

Coconut milk can actually improve your immune system. This is made from a combination of coconut water and cream mixed together.

166

Many people use this as a nondairy milk substitute.

We'll discuss coconut oil in the "Oils" section. It has many healthful properties that help it deserve its own section.

Vegetables

Adding vegetables to your diet is critical to good health. In this section we'll look at the veggies that provide you with the most when it comes to nutrition and health.

A diet high in vegetables will help you to maintain a healthy weight and prevent many diseases.

Spinach

Spinach is rich in antioxidants and contains folic acid. Its dark green color comes from all of the powerful nutrients it contains. It's also high in protein – something that might surprise you.

Spinach provides a source of vitamin A, K, magnesium, and Vitamin C.

These and other nutrients in it allow it to help you prevent heart disease, improve your vision, strengthen your bones, and have healthier skin.

It can also reduce the number of migraine headaches you experience.

Superfoods that Fight Chronic Fatigue
Syndrome

You can eat it raw or cooked, but it's best to eat it raw or only lightly steamed to get the most nutrition.

Kale

Kale is one of those vegetables that many people don't really know what to do with.

It's often used as a garnish to make your plate more beautiful, but it gets left behind on the plate instead of eaten to absorb its nutrients.

Kale is rich in calcium, iron, vitamins A, C, and K, and is full of beta-carotene.

It also contains phytochemicals that are known to fight disease.

It also has antioxidants in the form of flavonoids that help you to fight inflammation.

It can be used just like lettuce in a salad and can also be cooked as a side dish. Experiment with different herbs to make kale a family favorite.

Garlic

Garlic is one of the things you either love or hate, but many people appreciate the delicious flavor it ads to food.

Researchers in Germany have discovered the health benefits of garlic including its high content of antioxidants.

Garlic is known to help prevent heart disease and cancer. It also can help to slow the aging process. You can purchase garlic supplements, but it's always better to get it from your food.

Garlic can be added to many sauces, soups, and dips to help improve flavor and add to your good health.

Sweet Potatoes

While sweet potatoes are "sweet" they actually do magical things for your blood sugar.

Rather than raising your blood sugar, they actually lower it and help you to maintain healthy insulin levels.

The orange color tells you that you're getting vitamins and minerals. Sweet potatoes contain vitamins A and C and are a rich source of potassium.

And because they're so delicious you don't need to add a lot of butter or any sugar. Try adding some plain yogurt instead.

Superfoods that Fight Chronic Fatigue Syndrome

Broccoli

Broccoli is one of those veggies that gets overlooked because it's pretty common. However, it has many health benefits and is actually considered a superfood because of its nutritional content.

Broccoli contains a lot of beta-carotene which you usually expect to see in orange or red vegetables.

It's also high in vitamins A and C and contains fiber to help with heart health and good digestion.

There are many ways to eat broccoli and it has a pleasing flavor that most people enjoy. Just because it's common doesn't mean that it's not super!

Pumpkin

The autumn brings squash and pumpkins are actually a form of squash. And while they're fun to carve and decorate for Halloween, they actually are frequently overlooked as a superfood.

But pumpkins are full of fiber and potassium. They also contain magnesium and vitamin C as well as vitamin E.

They also contain carotenoids – a chemical in plants that's also an anti-inflammatory.

Roasting a pumpkin will help you to separate the meat from the skin. You can puree it or just season it and chop it up.

Oils

There are several different types of oils that you can incorporate into your diet that are considered superfoods because of all they provide for your body.

Olive Oil

Olive oil is perhaps one of the most well-known oils when it comes to reducing your risk of heart disease.

It helps your cholesterol to normalize and research has shown that it can protect your heart from damage.

Olive oil can be eaten in salad dressings and drizzled over vegetables. It can also be used for cooking because it can handle high heat.

You'll want to look for high quality extra virgin olive oil. This is oil that's pressed and produced without any added chemicals.

Coconut Oil

Coconut oil has become widely accepted as a superfood, in spite of the fact that it's a saturated fat.

But what you've heard about saturated fat isn't all true.

In fact, this oil is helpful for many health conditions including balancing your hormones, blood sugar, and your cells' ability to heal.

It also can help with weight loss and will help you to have healthy skin and hair.

It's a solid at room temperature, but can be melted and used for low temperature cooking or added to tea or a smoothie.

You'll want to make sure you look for extra virgin coconut oil that's produced organically to make sure you're not adding toxins to the body.

This is available in health food stores, but can even be found in major supermarkets now because of its recent popularity.

Fish Oil

Fish oil has become one of the most popular supplements recommended by physicians and dietitians. Fish oil has been shown to help lower bad cholesterol and improve good cholesterol.

It's also been shown to help with depression. In addition, the oil helps to nourish skin and treat problems such as eczema and psoriasis.

What's so wonderful about fish oil? For starters, it's an anti-inflammatory, so it helps with many conditions related to inflammation.

Secondly, it contains omega-3 fatty acids which are needed by the body, and the body can't produce them on its own.

Fish oil is a powerful supplement for protecting your heart. It's also thought to protect the nervous system and studies are being conducted to understand its effect on Alzheimer's prevention and stroke prevention.

In addition, it can help with women's health to treat painful menses, breast pain, and hormone imbalances.

It's also used to help with the prevention of obesity. This is a powerful supplement that has a broad range of effects.

It's important to check with your physician before you begin taking fish oil as a supplement because it might interact with other medications you're taking. This may require an adjustment in your prescription.

Grains

While many people have jumped onto the no-carb craze, whole grains are still an important part of the diet. And whole grains are a great source of many nutrients you need as well as fiber.

There are several grains that have become known as superfoods because of their nutrients and the way they support health. Some of these are in the category of ancient grains.

You may not recognize all of the grains discussed here, but a trip to your local health food store can help you to get familiar with them quickly.

Quinoa

Quinoa is a grain that's rich in protein. In fact, 12-18 percent of it is protein. It also includes all of the essential amino acids your body needs for proper protein production.

It's also gluten-free, so if you're allergic to gluten or have celiac disease, this is a safe grain to eat.

This grain also has a large concentration of unsaturated healthy fats that help to protect your heart health. It also has minerals such as copper, magnesium, and iron.

This grain is becoming more and more popular and you'll be able to find it in your local supermarket.

It's been shown to help reduce the risk of diabetes as well as support healthy weight management by allowing you to feel fuller for longer.

It's full of antioxidants which help your body to handle the toxins of the environment and prevent aging. Of all whole grains, quinoa is considered the healthiest.

If you've never tried this grain before, you'll find that its texture is similar to rice. It can be used like rice or pasta and is cooked in much the same way by boiling it in water. It makes a great side dish or even a good base for a main dish.

Oats

Oats have been popular since the late 1990s when research showed that eating foods made with oats could reduce your risk for heart disease.

Oat bran in particular was touted as a superfood, but new research shows oat bran isn't all it's cracked up to be.

Still, oats are very healthy foods that do have the ability to help lower your cholesterol because of the fiber that helps to clear cholesterol from your blood and keep it from becoming deposited on blood vessels.

Oats are a low calorie food that is high in fiber and protein. This is the combination you should look for in a health food.

They have minerals such as zinc, copper, and magnesium. They also contain phytonutrients – natural chemicals that are powerful disease preventers.

Another important factor to consider with oatmeal is that it's common and easy to find. You can go just about anywhere and order oatmeal from the menu. So if you're traveling and still want to keep healthy habits, this is a good choice.

Whole Wheat

You may be avoiding foods made with flour, but you may want to reconsider your decision and eliminate only certain kinds of flour. White flour is made from whole wheat that has been refined and much of the nutrition has been removed.

This is the flour that makes white bread, cakes, cookies, and crackers. It doesn't have much nutritional value, but it does cause your blood sugar to spike in unhealthy ways.

Whole wheat, on the other hand, offers a great deal of nutrition and is a healthy choice. Much like oats, whole wheat contains high amounts of fiber and is high in protein.

It also contains phytochemicals that prevent disease. Whole wheat can help your heart to be healthier and can actually prevent weight gain.

When it comes to wheat products, you'll need to be careful to check for "whole wheat".

Many people buy wheat bread or crackers thinking that it is whole wheat. These products may have some whole wheat, but can be largely made from white flour.

Look for products that are 100% whole wheat or whole grain to make the healthiest choices. You can also find whole wheat pasta which is more healthful than white pastas.

Amaranth

Amaranth, along with quinoa, spelt, and teff, is an ancient grain. This contains a high amount of protein and also contains some essential amino acids that help your body to build proteins.

It's also known to help strengthen immunity and ward off disease. It's also gluten free, so people who are allergic to gluten or are just trying to avoid it will be able to enjoy this grain.

It has a peppery flavor and is great to use in soups or sauces. You may have to hunt down this grain in a health food store if it's not available in your local supermarket.

Superfoods that Fight Chronic Fatigue
Syndrome

Spelt

Spelt is another in the category of ancient grain. It's similar to wheat, but has some differences.

It has a nutty flavor that is very similar to the flavor of wheat. It can be used to make breads and pastas in the same way wheat can be used.

This particular grain has been shown to be able to improve cholesterol levels because of its high fiber content.

Spelt is high in copper and zinc and is also high in manganese – all needed to perform essential functions in the body.

You can find whole spelt at your local natural foods store and you can often find breads and pastas made from spelt when you shop at those stores.

Teff

Teff is a very small grain that's packs a large nutritional punch. It's easily prepared by steaming, boiling, or baking. You can even eat it in its raw state.

You'll want to experiment with side dishes and main dishes that incorporate this grain.

This particular grain is helpful with managing your weight because of how it breaks down slowly in the body.

The high fiber content makes it beneficial for managing your weight, digestion, and blood sugar levels.

This grain is also rich in vitamin A, vitamin C, thiamin, and niacin.

These nutrients support a healthy immune system and healthy heart. This grain can be an important way to prevent heart disease and reduce your risk of cancer.

It's also very high in bone building calcium. If you're always searching for ways to incorporate calcium, one cup of teff provides 40 percent of the calcium you need each day.

Brown Rice

While white rice is a carbohydrate you'll want to avoid, brown rice is very healthy and is recommended for good digestion and a healthy metabolism. This is a whole grain that includes high fiber levels and is low in calories.

Brown rice contains what's known as resistant starch. This type of carbohydrate actually helps your body to burn more fat and calories. So if you're interested in weight loss, this is a good food to eat.

It also helps you to have better digestion and delivers vitamins and minerals to your body including B1, B2, and B6 which help you to have more energy and is especially essential for women.

Barley

Barley is an ancient grain that isn't as popular as it should be outside of the production of beer. It can be eaten as a cereal for your morning breakfast and can be used like rice for side and main dishes.

Barley is high in fiber and low in calories. It supports healthy digestion and a healthy weight.

It can actually help you to lower your cholesterol and prevent cancers if you eat it regularly.

In addition, it contains a form of vitamin E that's bioavailable (meaning your body can digest it easily) as well as niacin which protect your heart.

Dairy

Dairy is a food that many people eliminate when they're working to improve their diet.

But if you choose to eat dairy, there's one form of it in particular that can be beneficial to your body – yogurt.

Yogurt

Yogurt is cultured from bacteria that are healthy for the body. There are different bacteria used in various brands of yogurt. But these bacteria are healthy for your digestive system and can improve your regularity.

They also help to improve the way your immune system functions so you're better able to fight off disease. Many illnesses can be prevented by eating healthy bacteria that's found in yogurt.

When you choose to eat yogurt, you'll want to look for an organic yogurt that's all natural.

Fish

In general, fish is a healthy source of protein and healthy fats.

It's a great food to eat, but there are a couple of fish that provide the best health benefits. If you're going to choose to eat any fish, these are your best bets:

Sardines

Sardines are actually just small fish that are high in omega-3 oils. They're so healthy because they contain high levels of calcium, vitamin D, protein, and omega-3 fatty acids.

Eating sardines can actually help you to lower your risk of heart disease, lower your cholesterol, and help you to build strong bones.

Superfoods that Fight Chronic Fatigue Syndrome

Many people are turned off by the idea of eating sardines, but they are truly beneficial for your health and may just be an acquired taste if you're adventurous enough to give them a try.

Salmon

Salmon is another oily fish that is rich in omega-3 oils. They're known for helping to prevent heart disease and even cancer.

Many people enjoy the flavor of salmon, though it can be too fishy for some.

Salmon is widely available in most supermarkets and health food stores.

Many people are concerned about preparing fish at home for their family, but salmon is actually a quick and easy protein to prepare.

Nuts and Seeds

Nuts and seeds provide some of the most important sources of oils, fiber, and protein.

They're easy to add to dishes and even eat as a snack on their own. Most nuts are good choices, but the ones featured here are the best because of their nutritional value.

Before we talk too much about each one in detail, it's important to address a common concern people have about eating nuts. Many people shy away from nuts because they contain high percentages of fats.

The good news is that the fat in nuts is actually healthy fat that protects your heart from disease.

Nuts are high in calories, but they help you to feel satisfied and give you a great source of protein. Don't be afraid to enjoy them dailyl.

Sesame Seeds

You may think of sesame seeds as just a topping for crackers or hamburger buns, but sesame seeds deserve to be more than an afterthought.

Sesame seeds contain lignans, important nutrients that help to control blood cholesterol.

By eating more sesame seeds you can work to maintain a healthy cholesterol level.

In turn, you'll be working to prevent heart disease and stroke that are often related to cholesterol deposits on blood vessel walls.

Sesame seeds are also high in vitamin E and can help to reduce inflammation in the body and slow down the aging process.

They also help to prevent cancer and lower blood pressure. Make sure to sprinkle a few on your meals each day.

Walnuts

Walnuts are tree nuts that are grown all over the world. They contain the most antioxidants of any nut, so they make a great choice for snacks or adding nuts to breads and cereals.

They're also high in omega-3 fatty acids which are beneficial for heart health.

They are high in vitamin E, folic acid, and zinc. All of these nutrients help with disease prevention and wellness.

Walnuts can be eaten raw or toasted and can be added to many different dishes.

The next time you feel a little hungry, grab a handful of walnuts for a healthy snack that satisfies.

Flaxseed

In recent years flaxseed has gained popularity as an important food for digestive health and heart health. Flaxseed is a great addition to smoothies, cereals, yogurt, or sauces to help add fiber.

Whole flaxseeds can't be broken down by the body, so in order to get the benefits you'll need to make sure and grind the seeds. You can buy them ground or grind them in a blender and store in the refrigerator.

The oil in flaxseeds is so beneficial for your body that it won't ever be stored as fat.

It's used to help keep your nervous system healthy, give you healthy skin and hair, and protect your heart from disease.

Eating one or two tablespoons of flaxseed each day with plenty of water will help your digestive system to stay regular.

This helps with weight loss and with cancer prevention. Flaxseed has a mild, nutty flavor that adds to many dishes without being overpowering.

Hemp seeds

Hemp seeds contain all the essential amino acids that your body needs to build structures and repair cells.

These seeds come from the cannabis plant, but don't contain any mind altering properties because they don't contain THC like marijuana.

They can be eaten raw or ground and added to other foods in the same way flaxseeds are eaten. Like many other seeds, hemp seeds have been found to help lower cholesterol.

185

They also provide a complete protein so they're really wonderful if you're a vegetarian and looking for good sources of protein.

They also provide your body with vitamin E, omega-3 fatty acids, magnesium, iron, and zinc.

You can eat the seeds or look for product such as hemp butter or hemp milk made from them. A natural foods store will carry many options.

Sunflower seeds

Sunflower seeds are a delicious treat that many people enjoy. But you may not know that this common snack has so many amazing health benefits.

These seeds are high in vitamins and healthy fats that help you to prevent disease.

They contain plant sterols that help to lower cholesterol levels naturally.

They also have anti-inflammatory properties that help to protect your body from heart disease, cancer, and chronic disease.

You'll also get an extra dose of iron and selenium when you eat sunflower seeds.

They're great eaten on their own, but also make a tasty addition to salads or yogurt. Eating them raw will give you the best benefit.

Almonds

Almonds are delicious and packed full of nutrition. Like many nuts, they contain healthy oils that help to keep cholesterol under control and protect you from heart disease.

They're also high in magnesium and vitamin E and these two nutrients help to further protect the heart.

Many healthcare providers recommend eating a handful of almonds each day to get a dose of healthy oils and nutrients.

They can be eaten raw or toasted. You can buy them whole, sliced, or slivered. They're wonderful in breads, main dishes, and salads.

Chia Seeds

When you hear the word "chia" you may think of the beloved Chia Pet statues that grow hair or fur from seed. But those little seeds that turn into sprouts on your garden statue actually have nutritional value.

Chia seeds actually have more omega-3 and omega-6 fatty acids than flax seeds. They also contain vitamin B, calcium, potassium, and are high in fiber.

Because they're high in fiber, they help to regulate blood sugar levels which prevents weight gain and can help to prevent diabetes.

Superfoods that Fight Chronic Fatigue
Syndrome

It's important to soak chia seeds before eating them. You should soak 1/8 cup of chia seeds in one cup of water overnight so that your body will be able to digest them properly. They naturally absorb a lot of water, so eating them dry can actually cause constipation.

To the soaked seeds you can add fruit, honey, and chopped nuts in order to make a delicious cereal for a meal.

Unlike flax seeds, chia seeds don't need to be ground up in order to digest them.

However, if you have trouble with digestion and irregularity you may want to grind them first.

Peanuts

Peanuts are commonly eaten and used for peanut butter all over the world. Many people have avoided peanuts because of concerns about fat, but peanuts are actually very healthful.

When it comes to peanut butter, you need to be discerning. Many peanut butter products are full of sugar, hydrogenated oils, and other additives that counteract the nutrition of peanuts.

When you're shopping for peanut butter look for natural peanut butter that only contains peanuts and maybe salt.

This type of peanut butter usually has a layer of oil covering the top. You'll need to stir it and refrigerate to keep the oil from settling.

Peanuts contain healthy oils that help you to keep your heart healthy and can even help you with weight loss.

They also contain antioxidants which will help you to prevent cancer and other diseases.

These tasty nuts are also high in fiber and support healthy digestion. You can enjoy peanuts as a standalone snack or you can add them to salads and other dishes. Peanut butter is perfect paired with a piece of fruit.

Herbs and Spices

Herbs and spices can provide you with many nutrients when used regularly.

They can also help add flavor to a healthy diet. Many herbs and spices have healthy benefits, but these are some of the best.

Turmeric

Turmeric comes from the root of the turmeric plant. It's full of antioxidants which provide it with the yellow color.

It also helps the body to maintain stable blood sugar levels. This helps with both maintaining a healthy weight and preventing diabetes.

This herb also helps to protect your heart and brain from inflammation reducing your risk of heart disease and dementia.

It can also help to reduce inflammation that causes eczema and psoriasis of the skin. It also improves acne.

You'll also find that eating turmeric often can help you to have a stronger immune system and less joint pain. In addition, it can be used to help menstrual problems for women.

The flavor of turmeric is tart and sometimes bitter. It's used often in Southeast Asian cuisine.

But at home you can add it to just about any dish. It's wonderful in soups, with poultry and fish, and in grain dishes.

Oregano

Oregano is a delicious Mediterranean herb that's used widely in Italian and Greek cuisine.

It contains beta-carotene, copper, niacin, and many antioxidants. It prevents damage to cells and helps cell to repair damage.

Using oregano regularly can be particularly helpful in preventing cancer, heart disease, and inflammatory illnesses.

It can also help to reduce the growth of bad bacteria in the gut, protecting you from bowel problems.

Oregano is delicious in many different dishes and sauces. It's best to eat fresh oregano. Oregano can be grown easily in an indoor herb garden or in your outdoor garden.

Cinnamon

Cinnamon is one of the most beloved spices used for baking and adding a comforting flavor to foods. But what you may not know is that cinnamon is very powerful when it comes to maintaining a healthy blood sugar.

This can really help to reduce the effects of type II diabetes and even be part of the solution to reverse its effects. Cinnamon grows most common in China and Vietnam, but you can find it in almost any supermarket.

You should aim to eat a teaspoon of cinnamon each day - which can be eaten in teas, sprinkled on fruits, or added to other dishes. You can also purchase cinnamon supplements if you don't like the flavor of it.

Superfoods that Fight Chronic Fatigue Syndrome

Ginger

Ginger is a root that's commonly used to flavor Asian foods. It can be added to stir fry, salad dressings, and marinades for meats and vegetables. You'll want to use fresh ginger root that can be found in the produce section of the store.

Ginger can be used to prevent many types of cancer because it contains antioxidants.

It's also used as a natural way to treat nausea and stomach upset. If you suffer from motion sickness, ginger can help to calm your stomach.

This root also helps to kill bacteria either internally or on your skin. It can also kill parasites that make it into the body.

It also increases circulation in the body and is thought to be an aphrodisiac.

Cayenne Pepper

If you like spicy foods, you're probably familiar with cayenne pepper. This is a spicy pepper that's used in many foods. Not only does it have a delicious flavor that adds heat to a dish, it also has health benefits.

Cayenne pepper is actually helpful for treating problems with stomach inflammation and digestive problems, though it may seem like a spicy pepper would do just the opposite. It also helps to clear your sinuses and help you to breathe properly.

In addition, it prevents heart disease and helps maintain vascular health. If you're experiencing joint pain, cayenne pepper can bring relief and it can relieve headaches as well.

If you enjoy the flavor and heat, you can eat cayenne peppers as part of your meals.

But if that's a bit much for you, you can also take cayenne supplements that give you the health benefits without the burning tongue.

Black Pepper

Just below salt, black pepper is one of the most common seasonings used for food. But it also contains nutrients that help you to have better health.

It contains capsaicin, piperine, and gingerol compounds that actually work to speed your metabolism.

Black pepper is also an anti-inflammatory which is critical to the prevention of disease and can bring relief to CFS and other conditions such as arthritis.

It helps to prevent heart disease and stroke as well.

So when it's time for your next meal, sprinkle a little extra pepper on your plate.

Miscellaneous

There are a few superfoods that don't fit into the other categories mentioned here. They help to provide health benefits for people with CFS and support general wellness.

Green Tea

Many people are experiencing the benefits of drinking green tea. This tea is made from unfermented tea leaves rather than fermented leaves used for black tea. This helps to preserve the nutrients in the tea leaves.

Green tea contains antioxidants that help to prevent disease and reduce inflammation.

It also helps to maintain a healthy metabolism and can aid any weight loss efforts. Instead of having a morning cup of coffee, try switching to a cup of green tea.

To get the most benefit from your tea consumption, it's a good idea to drink two or three cups each day.

It's best to drink it hot rather than in cold drinks. However, make sure it's not so hot that it burns your mouth and throat.

Dark Chocolate

Many people are happy and surprised to find out that dark chocolate is actually a health food. But before you get too carried away, you only need to eat a small piece each day to get the benefits.

Dark chocolate has a higher concentration of cacao than milk chocolate. That cacao is where all the health benefits arise.

This type of chocolate helps to lower blood pressure and prevent heart disease. It may also help to prevent damage to blood vessels from hardened arteries.

You'll want to eat a piece that's equal to or less than 100 calories each day. That's enough to give you the benefits without causing you to gain weight from the indulgent food.

Bee pollen and Honey

The hard work of bees is very beneficial for humans. Bee pollen is actually the food that very young bees eat in the hive.

This food is high in protein and provides many nutrients that nourish a young bee and can help you to experience good health.

Superfoods that Fight Chronic Fatigue Syndrome

Bee pollen helps to prevent bacteria from growing and can be used as an antibiotic.

It also helps to keep cholesterol levels normal and specifically can raise HDL (the good cholesterol).

This amazing food can also be used to treat infertility in women and reduce allergies. It can also help you to manage a healthy weight.

When you eat bee pollen granules, make sure you don't cook them as it will destroy the nutrients. It can be added to salad dressings, toast, and added to juices.

Honey is another product from bees that has aids in good health. This is especially true if you consume raw honey which can be found at most natural food stores and some supermarkets.

Honey contains antioxidants that can prevent cancer and slow the aging process.

It also can help to provide you with relief from allergies that cause coughing and sneezing. If you want to try natural methods to deal with allergies, honey is a great choice.

This delicious substance also helps to fight bacteria and can reduce your risk of bacterial infections. It can also be used on top of the skin to kill bacteria and promote healing.

Water

Water is the most important substance you can put into your body. Unfortunately with the advent of sodas, many people don't get enough water. You want to make sure you're drinking at least eight to ten glasses of water daily.

This helps to flush toxins from the body and provide the necessary fluid for water soluble vitamins to be broken down. Hydration also helps you to have more lubrication in your joints and your skin.

While technically not a "food", water is an important substance that shouldn't be overlooked when you're paying attention to good nutrition and superfoods.

Your cells are made mostly of water and need a continual supply in order to function properly. Pay attention to your water drinking habits and make sure you're getting enough.

Eating A Raw Food Diet

There are many benefits of eating superfoods especially as an integral part of a raw food diet. Eating food that is unprocessed and as close as possible to its natural state has become very popular in recent years.

One reason for the health benefits of raw food is that it helps to reduce inflammation in your system which is often a debilitating health issue for the body to deal with.

Is Inflammation Making You Ill?

A Raw Food Diet Could Be the Cure

Inflammation in and of itself is not always a bad thing. It's your body's natural response to dealing with foreign invaders. You need acute episodes of inflammation in specific areas to help fight infection.

For example, if you cut your finger you'll notice that it's red and tender for a few days while it's healing. During that time the immune system has sent many different cells to the area to help keep infection out of the body and to heal the skin.

But that type of inflammation doesn't hang around for a very long time unless you have a very serious injury. In general, you notice the area for a few days and then it's gone and things are back to normal. This is a good and healthy process.

The problem is when inflammation becomes a chronic condition. This is when inflammation gets turned on, but doesn't get turned off. As a result you can have all kinds of chronic health problems related to the inflammatory process.

What Illnesses Are Related to Inflammation?

Many illnesses have been found to be related to chronic inflammation. While alternative medicine practitioners have recognized inflammation as a problem for many years, the rest of the medical community only recently caught on to this detrimental problem.

As more reach has been conducted, many diseases have been linked to inflammation. Some examples include:

Fibromyalgia
Chronic fatigue syndrome
Arthritis
Diabetes
Parkinson's disease
Alzheimer's disease
Depression
Osteoporosis
Irritable bowel syndrome
Cancer
Hardening of the arteries
Eczema

And more and more are being linked to this problem. The good news is that with a greater understanding of what causes this inflammation, it's possible to make lifestyle changes to improve it.

Superfoods that Fight Chronic Fatigue Syndrome

Benefits of Eating Raw

Because you won't be using heat to prepare foods, your body will be able to take full advantage of the nutrients in your food. And getting good nutrition through your diet is always better than taking a pill.

The chemistry of food shows us that nutrients are in their most bioavailable form when they're in the original plant, rather than being extracted and made into a supplement. It's not that taking a supplement is bad; it's just not as effective as good nutrition.

Unfortunately, the typical modern diet of someone living in an industrialized country is terribly unhealthy and leads to problems with chronic inflammation. Many experts believe that the prevalence of chronic disease is directly related to diet.

When you're constantly putting "junk" into the body, the immune system works in overdrive to help clear it. But in the process, the chronic inflammation causes more problems.

Helping Your Body to Heal

With the raw food diet, you don't need to rely on medications produced in a lab to subdue inflammation. In fact, the real cure is to change your diet so that your body's natural healing systems can do their jobs.

Medications may help short-term, but they themselves can be processed as toxins by the body. It puts strain on the liver, kidneys, and other organs to take medication chronically. And anti-inflammatory medications can be hard on the digestive system.

The raw food diet allows you to get all of the good nutrition you need. It also gives your body the chance to turn off the immune response that's causing your problems. Then inflammation will be reserved for acute times when it's needed most.

When this inflammation is reversed, you'll find that your risk of cancer, diabetes, heart disease, and mental illness will decrease. You'll also have more energy, clearer skin, and fewer aches and pains.

The raw food diet is a prescription for soothing your body and allowing it to enjoy good health and total wellness, so it is well worth your time to learn more about superfoods and eating raw foods as much as possible in your CFS diet.

You can learn more about the benefits of eating raw here: http://www.learn-how-to-do-it.com/how-to-start-raw-food-diet.html and Helene Malmsio has also written a book detailing how to begin with the transition to a raw food diet that is available in bookstores and online outlets:

http://www.amazon.com/gp/product/B00AQY0BZY "The Raw Food Diet Made Simple - Transitioning to a Raw Food Plan for Better Health, Vibrant Energy, and Weight Loss" which can be read as either kindle or paperback format.

Conclusion
- Handling Your Recovery

After having a health problem for so long there is a mental aspect to this that needs to be addressed.

When you are not well with chronic fatigue syndrome then you have good days when you can almost feel normal and bad days when the world is almost too much to bear.

When you begin to recover this cycling of good and bad days does not stop.

We often see people who have been sick and had no answers for the longest time who get on a nutrition therapy program and then one day wake up feeling fantastic.

They have energy, they do not have pain, and they actually slept and are now refreshed. It can feel almost miraculous.

Conclusion

Actually it is miraculous but it the miracle of the body healing itself to function the way it is designed to function.

While this seems really good there is a danger here.

There is a huge temptation to do things in excess, to clean house, to do the jobs that have been waiting until you have the energy one day, or to just get out and do things with friends and family that you have been unable to do until now.

That is great, but too often people overdo it.

Next day they wake up feeling they are right back where they were! The spark of energy is no longer there, they did too much the day before, now they are tired, often they have muscle pain, and it can seem that they are worse than they were before.

It feels like you have been given a present and then had it snatched away.

If you are not prepared for this you can lose heart and it can even trigger a day of depression.

You need to understand this up front.

You have been having good days and bad days.

You will keep on having good days and bad days.

When you get a great day then give thanks to God and treat yourself with care and respect.

Allow the process to take its course.

What we can tell you is that when this begins to work with you then there will be more good days. There will still be bad days. You will still over-estimate your capacity and occasionally crash and burn from over exertion.

Over time though you will find that the good days get better and the bad days are not as bad. The time comes when the bad days are still better than the previous old good days used to be.

It took a long time to get to the bottom of your health problems and recovery is not going to happen overnight.

Be patient.

It is a really good idea to *take a snapshot* of where you are now. Create a benchmark that you can measure future progress against.

What we mean is for you to write down everything that is wrong with you right now; the food allergies, the bowel problems, the split hair and the nails that shatter, your poor skin condition, your concentration issues, the colds and flu you catch, the yeast and Candida infections, the hormonal issues. Write down everything.

Conclusion

Then, when you have a day that you think you are slipping back to where you were before, you can pull out this list and look though it and you will be amazed and encouraged by just how far you have come and how well things really are going.

It is all too easy to begin taking for granted the new health improvements as you go along each day, month after month. Sometimes it's the littlest thing that will bring back the memories of 'the bad old days' and surprise you to realize how much your health and energy and stamina levels have improved.

It is a step-by-step process, and it will also require many lifestyle changes, learning to pace yourself, and getting access to whatever self-help therapies you can put in your tool box for your road to recovery and maintenance.

There are many happy stories of people we know who have beaten their CFS and others who have at least learned how to control and manage their severe conditions.

One case that comes to mind immediately with full blown CFS is Carlene S. who lives in our countryside region of Australia as well.

She was a primary teacher and bringing up children on a rural property.

As her CFS became worse she tried to just live with it. She talked with every medical professional and

206

specialist and nutritional consultant she could find and tried everything but nothing worked for her. Eventually she found that she could not continue with her teaching.

She was finding that she do a story for the children during their quiet time only to be woken up herself by teachers from other rooms who had come in to find out what all the noise was about. She was falling asleep herself and the kids were running riot.

Eventually she was only getting out of bed about 2 hours a day as she just did not have energy to do more.

After being on the recommended nutritional therapy program for a few months she turned around her health and went on to home-school all her children and to run her little farm.

She works much too hard with the children and the farm but she says that she just loves it and she gives thanks to God every day that she has energy now to do the things that she does.

The point here is that CFS can develop in to a life crushing condition but that even then it can be turned around and that you can get back to living, and enjoying, a normal life.

Conclusion

The information we have shared with you in Volume 1 and 2 in this series are our attempt to give you the tools to rebuild your health and to be able to make informed decisions and choices about the lifestyle and nutritional changes that will help you achieve lifelong health and wellness.

We appreciate you investing your time in reading this book and hope that you have found the answers that will help you to join us to beat CFS with the use of self help lifestyle strategies, nutrition and natural supplements.

Our personal experiences have helped us both to manage our own conditions for over 20 years now and to help others overcome their health challenges.

If you have more unanswered questions you are invited to arrange for a personal private (no obligation) consultation with Warren Tattersall. He can be contacted on the form at his site: http://www.thehealthsuccesssite.com/contact-us.html and he will be happy to discuss his recommendations with you in person.

If you would like to learn more about the specific CFT Treatments and self help Therapies discussed briefly in this book, just check out Volume One in this series here: http://www.amazon.com/Beat-Chronic-Fatigue-Syndrome-ebook/dp/B00ANM51XG

"How to Beat Chronic Fatigue Syndrome...and get your life back!"

Remember That Things Will Get Better!

When you're in the beginning or middle of your struggles with CFS it can seem like there's no light at the end of the tunnel. But learning from our experiences and from those of others with CFS that we have helped, there will be a time when things get better for you.

Discouragement can keep you from taking action and make you feel helpless. If you've learned anything by reading the suggestions here, we hope that you've learned that you have a lot of power over your own health and that you can make things better.

It won't happen all at once and it won't happen overnight, but gradually as you learn your own body's triggers and what works for you, you'll gain more energy and start to feel better each day.

We expect that if you follow the guidelines we have given in this book you will be able to clear away the symptoms of your CFS and be able to live a healthy active lifestyle.

With the understanding of how your body works that you have gathered from your own experience and added to from this book we expect that you will be

209

able to monitor your own condition and will not relapse into CFS again.

We wish you well on your personal journey to better health and would love to hear from you about your personal story in recovering from CFS.

You can leave your comments or ask questions of the authors through the comments section at http://www.thehealthsuccesssite.com/Chronic-fatigue-syndrome.html

We want to thank you for purchasing *"Nutritional Therapy Guide for a CFS Diet – How to Eat Yourself Healthy Again!"*

We enjoyed putting this information together for you to give you an overview of Chronic Fatigue Syndrome and to let you get a broad brush picture of what you are dealing with as either a suffer or as a Carer of someone who has the condition.

We have endeavored to give you tools to understand your options in how to address your own situation and how to access support from medical and alternative health professionals.

We have made every effort to ensure the accuracy and completeness of the content provided in this book.

However, the authors or any other person associated with this book makes no warranties or guarantees, expressed or implied, regarding errors or omissions and assumes no legal liability or responsibility for loss or damage resulting from the use of information contained within.

Additionally, the author or associated persons do not guarantee, expressed or implied, for the accuracy, completeness, or usefulness of any information, apparatus, product, or process disclosed, or represents that its use would guarantee improvement or success in relation to subject written.

Any reference herein to any specific commercial products, process, or service by trade name, trademark, manufacturer, or otherwise, does not necessarily constitute or imply its endorsement, recommendation, or favoring.

The content of *"Nutritional Therapy Guide for a CFS Diet – How to Eat Yourself Healthy Again!"* is copyright protected, with all rights reserved and may not be copied or imitated in whole or part without first requesting and receiving full written permission from the author.

Again, thank you for allowing us to give you this overview on the condition of Chronic Fatigue Syndrome.

If you would like to visit:

Conclusion

http://www.thehealthsuccesssite.com/Chronic-fatigue-syndrome.html you can leave your comments and feedback on this book and ask any questions you may have about CFS in general.

Also we invite you to leave your review of this book at Amazon.

About the Authors:

Warren Tattersall

I had a problem with my own health that had plagued me for all of my life.

My elder and younger brothers had high energy levels and I had low energy. I didn't understand why, and I still cannot explain it, but it had been with me all my life and I lived with it.

As a schoolboy I had unexplained energy drop periods where I would just go to bed and sleep for 24 hours. Blood tests showed a drop in the red blood cells in that period but no-one could tell me anything about it.

In my 20's I went to a naturopath to ask about improving energy and she checked my diet and almost had a fit. She had me change my eating process dramatically. I did that for 90 days and it made no difference to the condition at all that I could see.

I had a Homeopathic consultation at one stage and religiously used the drops for a few months in the belief that I needed to stick to anything for at least 90 days. Again, it made not the slightest difference to the way I felt.

I tried a Chinese herbalist once. I figured that anything that tasted that bad HAD to be good for you but again, another 3 months and no energy improvement at all.

When I was going out with the girl who became my wife there was an occasion that I fell asleep while sitting at the table in a restaurant. This is an embarrassing thing at any time but when there are only the 2 of you there it is something that keeps being recalled in conversation for 20 years!!

In my early 30's I went to my General Practitioner and had a serious conversation with him because the periods of weariness seemed to be getting worse and I thought there should be _something_ that could be done.

I am 6 ft 2 in (187 cm) and he is much shorter than I am. He did all the blood tests and then patiently explained to me that I was tall and he was short. He did not like being short but there was nothing he could do about it. He said that he had high energy and I had low energy and that was just the way it was. Live with it!!

I'd lived with my 'condition' all my life and after that I pretty much accepted it and I did not really notice the effect of it in my world any more. I just accepted that I naturally had very low energy levels and that every 6 or 8 weeks I would have an energy drop out that would make normal living a big challenge for a few days, but I knew it would pass.

When I started to use nutritional supplement products it was just to see what it did and because it may be able to give me a benefit for my Martial Arts.

It was only 4 or 5 days later I remember standing at my wardrobe in the morning getting out a shirt and just freezing up. I realized that for the first time in my life I could not remember getting out of bed! I had never just woken up and just got out of bed.

Every day I used to come slowly to consciousness and then fought myself to get moving. This day I just woke up rested and alert. It was one of those moments that you remember forever.

On that day my energy lifted. I can't say it 'came back' because I could never remember having it in the first place. I can miss sleep and get just 4 or 5 hours for a couple of nights in a row and still do not have energy drop-outs during the day. When I do get really tired it is my own fault, but one night with 8 hours sleep and I am refreshed again.

Once I began incorporating these products into my CFS therapy I have not had to do much of anything else, apart from my daily use of nutrition supplements, which is now so engrained into my lifestyle that I do not even notice it.

This has lasted for 20 years now and someone asked me the other day what the side effects are of taking 'supplements' for extended times. In my own case I have an answer to that.

Earlier in the year I turned 57 and as a matter of good practice I occasionally get a full medical check (to be frank the results are always really good so I'm happy to do it).

This last test generated a call from the pathologist re the results and I was concerned that there might be a problem because I had not expected a call. He said that no, quite the reverse.

The results were really good, or at least they would be really good for someone in their mid 20's. He did not believe that results like these, which uniformly perfect across the full spectrum, were possible for someone in their mid 50's.

The point here is that whatever your personal beliefs may be about the benefits of taking daily supplements and vitamins, it cannot be denied that consistently eating healthy food and supplements has a very positive effect on your body in the long-term.

I think the summary of my own story is that you need to keep looking till you find the answer best suited for you, and when you get it right you can expect, God willing, to regain good health and keep it for decade after decade.

To ask Warren any questions about your condition, contact him here: http://www.thehealthsuccesssite.com/contact-us.html

Helene Malmsio

At 17 I was overworked and already anemic, when I contracted glandular fever in 1976. I thought it was just a bad flu and didn't get it treated until my throat was so sore that it was too painful to even take a normal breath.

I did finally get on a course of antibiotics, but did not support my recovery with supplements to help undo the damage of massive doses of antibiotics to my already compromised system, or improve my poor diet.

Sure enough, within a few years I found that I was chronically ill with every cold, flu, allergy, and joint pain that I had ever imagined possible.

Every morning I would wake up feeling like I had the worst Flu ever, multiplied by 10. I also felt a level of total exhaustion like nothing I had ever known before. It was totally bewildering to me.

In 1988 I was laughingly diagnosed with the 'Yuppie Flu' as it was known then, and told to just 'take some rest'. I was running my own business and my workload did not allow for any rest, and within 18 months I was totally incapacitated.

I was physically incapacitated to the point where I simply could not muster the energy or motivation to get out of bed, never mind to leave the house or go to the office, so I had to close my consulting business.

At one point I admit that I even became suicidal from my deep depression and the belief that I would never be able to have a normal life again. There was so much pain and hopelessness, there really did not seem to be anything to look forward to in life.

It required 12 months of bed rest and doing everything I could think of or learn about to help my recovery, before I could muster enough energy to try to participate in the workforce again. My partner at the time informed me that I was the most boring person he knew, because I always had to sleep for the entire weekend just to be able to go back to work again on Monday morning.

In 1991 I found a doctor specializing in CFS treatments who identified 6 common influenza strains in my blood that are known to trigger the illness, along with the initial GF. He said that he was surprised I was able to function at all, never mind be able to hold down a job, as my case was one of the most severe he had seen.

I was prescribed a 90 day CFS treatment program that included a range of dozens of bottles of Vega tested vitamins and minerals to take every day, with half a dozen oral allergy drops to build my immunity to these triggers also attacking my system.

And every week I endured an hour of an IV feeding a vitamin mix direct into my blood and organs. This treatment would then send my body into a state of shock for the rest of the day, with shivering and considerable pain throughout my entire body. And I achieved absolutely no relief from my CFS at the end of the long treatment program.

My doctor told me that I should just try undertaking another course of the same treatment. I felt shattered and hopeless again, as I simply could not endure another few months of that painful treatment.

About the Authors

But I was on a cause, and determined to get my life back. I kept researching and testing. And as a result of spending the last 25 years checking out every possible therapy I have ever heard of, I now know how to cope better with my CFS and how to recover from relapses when they happen.

As a result I now know how to pace myself, and how to deal with the cyclical relapses, what nutritional supplements work for me, and I still apply a combination of the therapies featured in this book for an individual CFS therapy plan that works for me.

Nowadays I am often even considered to be a 'dynamic' person by some people, and that is a testament to how well you can recover under the right circumstances.

My hope is that sharing this information in this book set will be of help to you and save you many years of experimenting and testing like I had to undergo. I really look forward to publishing more books in this series, as I believe you will get as much benefit as I have from learning every strategy to beat your CFS.